Advanced Techniques in the Management of Foot and Ankle Trauma

Editor

JUSTIN J. FLEMING

CLINICS IN PODIATRIC MEDICINE AND SURGERY

www.podiatric.theclinics.com

Consulting Editor
THOMAS J. CHANG

April 2018 • Volume 35 • Number 2

ELSEVIER

1600 John F. Kennedy Boulevard • Suite 1800 • Philadelphia, Pennsylvania, 19103-2899

http://www.theclinics.com

CLINICS IN PODIATRIC MEDICINE AND SURGERY Volume 35, Number 2
April 2018 ISSN 0891-8422, ISBN-13: 978-0-323-58324-4

Editor: Lauren Boyle
Developmental Editor: Sara Watkins

Clinics in Podiatric Medicine and Surgery (ISSN 0891-8422) is published quarterly by Elsevier Inc., 360 Park Avenue South, New York, NY 10010-1710. Months of issue are January, April, July, and October. Business and Editorial Offices: 1600 John F. Kennedy Blvd., Ste. 1800, Philadelphia, PA 19103-2899. Customer Service Office: 3251 Riverport Lane, Maryland Heights, MO 63043. Periodicals postage paid at New York, NY and additional mailing offices. Subscription prices are $294.00 per year for US individuals, $544.00 per year for US institutions, $100.00 per year for US students and residents, $382.00 per year for Canadian individuals, $657.00 for Canadian institutions, $439.00 for international individuals, $657.00 per year for international institutions and $220.00 per year for Canadian and foreign students/residents. To receive student/resident rate, orders must be accompanied by name of affiliated institution, date of term, and the *signature* of program/residency coordinator on institution letterhead. Orders will be billed at individual rate until proof of status is received. Foreign air speed delivery is included in all *Clinics* subscription prices. All prices are subject to change without notice. POSTMASTER: Send address changes to *Clinics in Podiatric Medicine and Surgery*, Elsevier Health Sciences Division, Subscription Customer Service, 3251 Riverport Lane, Maryland Heights, MO 63043. **Customer Service: 1-800-654-2452 (US). From outside of the US, call 314-447-8871. Fax: 314-447-8029. E-mail: JournalsCustomerService-usa@elsevier.com (for print support); JournalsOnlineSupport-usa@elsevier.com (for online support).**

Reprints. For copies of 100 or more of articles in this publication, please contact the Commercial Reprints Department, Elsevier Inc., 360 Park Avenue South, New York, NY 10010-1710. Tel.: 212-633-3874; Fax: 212-633-3820; E-mail: reprints@elsevier.com.

Clinics in Podiatric Medicine and Surgery is covered in *MEDLINE/PubMed (Index Medicus) and EMBASE/Excerpta Medica.*

Contributors

CONSULTING EDITOR

THOMAS J. CHANG, DPM
Clinical Professor and Past Chairman, Department of Podiatric Surgery, California College of Podiatric Medicine, Faculty, The Podiatry Institute, Redwood Orthopedic Surgery Associates, Santa Rosa, California

EDITOR

JUSTIN J. FLEMING, DPM
Director, Foot and Ankle Training Aria Jefferson Health System, Director, Philadelphia Foot and Ankle Trauma Fellowship, Fellow, American College of Foot and Ankle Surgeons, Faculty, Podiatry Institute, Newtown, Pennsylvania

AUTHORS

MICHAEL CALDERONE, DPM
Premier Orthopaedics, Kennett Square, Pennsylvania

FRANCESCA M. CASTELLUCCI-GARZA, DPM, MS
Resident, Departments of Orthopedics and Podiatry, Kaiser San Francisco Bay Area Foot and Ankle Residency Program, Kaiser Permanente Oakland Medical Center, Oakland, California

J. RANDOLPH CLEMENTS, DPM
Director of Podiatric Medical and Surgical Residency Education, Associate Professor of Orthopaedic Surgery, The Virginia Tech Carilion School of Medicine and Research Institute, Roanoke, Virginia

FRANÇOIS DIJOUR, DPM, PGY-2
Resident, Podiatric Medical and Surgical Residency, Reconstructive Rearfoot and Ankle, Carilion Clinic, Roanoke, Virginia

MICHAEL W. DOWNEY, DPM
Fellowship Trained Trauma & Reconstruction Foot/Ankle Surgeon, Trinity Foot & Ankle Specialists, Fort Worth, Texas

MATTHEW D. DOYLE, DPM, MS
Resident, Departments of Orthopedics and Podiatry, Kaiser San Francisco Bay Area Foot and Ankle Residency Program, Kaiser Permanente Oakland Medical Center, Oakland, California

JUSTIN J. FLEMING, DPM
Director, Foot and Ankle Training Aria Jefferson Health System, Director, Philadelphia Foot and Ankle Trauma Fellowship, Fellow, American College of Foot and Ankle Surgeons, Faculty, Podiatry Institute, Newtown, Pennsylvania

GRAHAM A. HAMILTON, DPM, FACFAS
Attending Staff, Foot and Ankle Surgery, Department of Podiatric Surgery, Palo Alto Foundation Medical Group, Dublin, California

KWASI Y. KWAADU, DPM, FACFAS
Assistant Professor, Department of Surgery, Temple University School of Podiatric Medicine, Philadelphia, Pennsylvania

TED C. LAI, DPM
Fellowship Trained Foot and Ankle Surgeon, Shore Orthopaedic University Associates, Somers Point, New Jersey

WESLEY LEONG, DPM, PGY-2
Resident, Podiatric Medical and Surgical Residency, Reconstructive Rearfoot and Ankle, Carilion Clinic, Roanoke, Virginia

SPENCER J. MONACO, DPM
Premier Orthopaedics, Kennett Square, Pennsylvania

RYAN B. RIGBY, DPM, FACFAS
Attending Physician, Logan Regional Orthopedics, Logan, Utah

RYAN T. SCOTT, DPM, FACFAS
Attending Physician, CORE Institute, Phoenix, Arizona

Contents

Foreword: Advanced Techniques in the Management of Foot and Ankle Trauma ix

Thomas J. Chang

Preface: Advanced Techniques in the Management of Foot and Ankle Trauma xi

Justin J. Fleming

Surgical Management Navicular and Cuboid Fractures 145

J. Randolph Clements, François Dijour, and Wesley Leong

The tarsal navicular is a critical component of the foot's medial longitudinal arch. Injuries to the navicular have significant long-term functional consequences. In addition to stress fractures, acute injuries to the navicular include acute avulsion, tuberosity, and body fractures. Nonoperative treatment is the mainstay for avulsion injuries and nondisplaced body fractures. Open reduction and internal fixation is performed to achieve anatomic reduction in the other situations. Common complications following operative intervention include pain, stiffness, posttraumatic arthritis, avascular necrosis, nonunion, and hindfoot deformity. This article provides an overview for the recognition and treatment of common presentations of these injuries as described in the literature.

Management of Talar Fractures 161

Kwasi Y. Kwaadu

Fractures of the talus are significant injuries with associated significant complications where the recovery zenith is less frequently good to excellent and more commonly fair to satisfactory. These outcomes are a consequence of combinations of the inherent intrinsic and surrounding anatomy, technical and logistic difficulties in adequate fracture access, and the high-energy mechanisms typically associated with these injuries that further traumatize the surrounding tissues. This article reviews and provides current management recommendations for these devastating injuries.

Paradigm Shift for the Surgical Management of Calcaneal Fractures? 175

Spencer J. Monaco, Michael Calderone, and Justin J. Fleming

Calcaneal fractures account for up to 75% of all foot fractures and 1% to 2% of all fractures. Approximately 75% of calcaneal fractures are intraarticular, resulting in a prolonged recovery, more pain, and disability. The most common mechanism of injury includes falls from a height and motor vehicle accidents. This article reviews studies that compare nonoperative with operative treatment. The literature continues to support surgical intervention; however, these injuries can still be managed nonoperatively in certain clinical scenarios. This article focuses on the surgical management of intraarticular calcaneal fractures and highlights the sinus tarsi approach.

Role for Primary Repair of Deltoid Ligament Complex in Ankle Fractures 183

Ryan B. Rigby and Ryan T. Scott

Acute deltoid injuries may occur with ankle fractures. They are often left to heal without repair, possibly leading to chronic medial ankle instability. Stress radiographs identify the need for surgical repair of fractures or soft tissue damage. Gravity stress views have benefits over manually stressing the ankle. MRI can explore the extent of medial soft tissue injuries. Arthroscopy can evaluate and potentially treat deltoid injuries. Interposition of the deltoid may preclude adequate fracture reduction. Except with deltoid tear, fractures should be reduced and fixated, then the deltoid assessed. With persistent instability, primary repair may prevent long-term sequelae.

Arthroscopic-Assisted Open Reduction Internal Fixation 199

Graham A. Hamilton, Matthew D. Doyle, and Francesca M. Castellucci-Garza

The indications for arthroscopy have expanded over the years. Arthroscopic-assisted open reduction internal fixation in the setting of acute trauma is gaining popularity with foot and ankle surgeons. It serves to facilitate direct visualization of fracture fragments and allows for precise articular reduction with minimal soft tissue insult. Current evidence reports a high incidence of chondral injury with ankle fractures. Arthroscopy performed at the time of open reduction internal fixation allows for joint inspection and potential treatment of these posttraumatic defects.

Minimally Invasive Plate Osteosynthesis for Distal Tibia Fractures 223

Ted C. Lai and Justin J. Fleming

Surgical treatment of distal tibia fractures can present as a difficult task. Intramedullary nailing (IMN), external fixation, and open reduction internal fixation (ORIF) have displayed various complications ranging from a high rate of knee morbidity with IMN to wound complications and infection with ORIF. Minimally invasive plate osteosynthesis (MIPO) has been used to decrease development of these complications. MIPO respects the soft tissue envelope along with maintaining the biological environment needed for proper osseous healing. Favorable results have been shown with MIPO in regard to function, healing time, and decreased complications.

Primary Arthrodesis in Severely Comminuted Fractures 233

Michael W. Downey, Ted C. Lai, and Justin J. Fleming

At present there is controversy regarding the appropriate treatment of severely comminuted fractures of the lower extremity. Even with near-perfect anatomic reduction of severely comminuted fractures, development of posttraumatic arthritis is still present at an increased rate. Primary fusion of comminuted fractures of the foot and ankle creates successful and predictable outcomes, which dismisses the chance of developing posttraumatic arthritis and decreases complications and the need for revisional procedures.

Intramedullary Nailing of Fibular Fractures **259**

Justin J. Fleming

The reamed intramedullary (IM) technique has many benefits. However, open plating is the most commonly used technique. Previously, IM stabilization was reserved for fibular fractures, which were given lower priority, and generally associated with injuries to the distal tibia or instances in which the soft tissue envelope was unsuitable for an open approach. This article reviews the literature and the level of evidence and presents case examples and operative technique.

CLINICS IN PODIATRIC MEDICINE AND SURGERY

FORTHCOMING ISSUES

July 2018
Use of Biologics for Foot and Ankle Surgery
Adam Landsman, *Editor*

October 2018
Innovations in Foot and Ankle Surgery
Guido A. LaPorta, *Editor*

January 2019
Perioperative Considerations in the Surgical Patient
Jeffrey Shook, *Editor*

RECENT ISSUES

January 2018
New Technologies in Foot and Ankle Surgery
Stephen A. Brigido, *Editor*

October 2017
Surgical Advances in Ankle Arthritis
Alan Ng, *Editor*

July 2017
Foot and Ankle Arthrodesis
John J. Stapleton, *Editor*

RELATED INTEREST

Foot and Ankle Clinics, March 2017 (Vol. 22, Issue 1)
Current Controversies in Foot and Ankle Trauma
Michael P. Swords, *Editor*
Available at: http://www.foot.theclinics.com/

Foreword

Advanced Techniques in the Management of Foot and Ankle Trauma

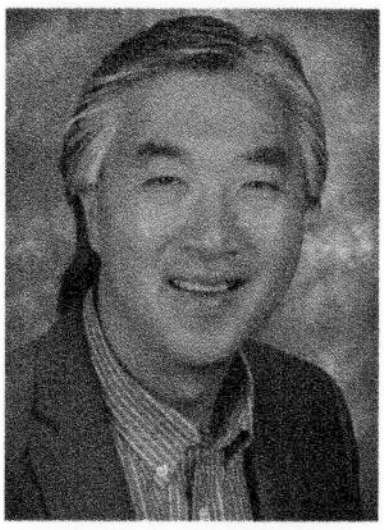

Thomas J. Chang, DPM
Consulting Editor

I hope you enjoyed the first *Clinics in Podiatric Medicine and Surgery* issue of 2018 on "New Technologies in Foot and Ankle Surgery," by Stephen A. Brigido. When I decided to have an issue centered on recent trauma updates as the second issue for 2018, my choice of an editor was relatively easy. Justin J. Fleming has published extensively on trauma topics and has established himself as a thought leader in lower-extremity trauma. I give recognition to Drs Jack Schuberth and George Gumann, who have both inspired and paved the way for many of our colleagues who now assume similar roles in management of lower-extremity trauma in their own communities. It is a trend that will only increase as training and experience grows.

I applaud Dr Fleming's efforts in gathering a list of pertinent topics and experienced authors. They have spent valuable time to further our education. These topics help define the quality and level of lower-extremity trauma management in 2018.

Enjoy this second 2018 issue of *Clinics in Podiatric Medicine and Surgery* on "Advanced Techniques in the Management of Foot and Ankle Trauma."

Thomas J. Chang, DPM
Redwood Orthopedic Surgery Associates
208 Concourse Boulevard
Santa Rosa, CA 95403, USA

E-mail address:
thomaschang14@comcast.net

Clin Podiatr Med Surg 35 (2018) ix
https://doi.org/10.1016/j.cpm.2018.01.002

Preface

Advanced Techniques in the Management of Foot and Ankle Trauma

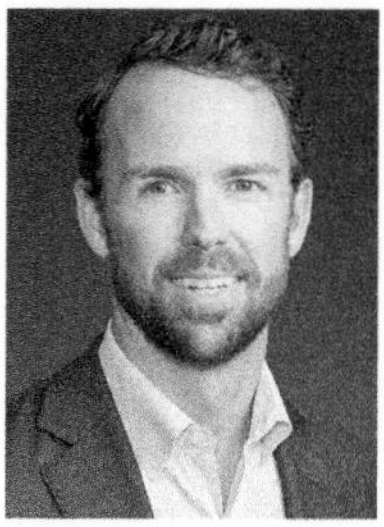

Justin J. Fleming, DPM
Editor

It is my pleasure to present this issue of *Clinics in Podiatric Medicine and Surgery* on "Advanced Techniques in the Management of Foot and Ankle Trauma." I had the distinct privilege of working with some very great people, who happen to be talented surgeons and thought leaders in our profession. We've included emerging areas of interest and debate, such as the importance of acute deltoid ligament repair, and newer techniques, such as intramedullary fixation of fibular fractures. I would like to personally thank the authors for the time, energy, and expertise that they put into this issue.

I'd like to dedicate this special issue to a mentor of mine named George Gumann. George provided me with a solid foundation in the management of foot and ankle fractures at Martin Army Community Hospital in Fort Benning, Georgia. I consider myself to be quite lucky to have learned from many incredible teachers, such as John Ruch, Alan Banks, and Craig Camasta; however, I attribute any success I may have had as a fracture surgeon to the wisdom imparted to me by George. He was a pioneer in our profession, whom many of us benefited, and continue to benefit, from. In the operating room, he was a perfectionist with an impeccable attention to detail. I find myself passing on the same principles to residents and fellows that he taught me 15 years ago.

Clin Podiatr Med Surg 35 (2018) xi–xii
https://doi.org/10.1016/j.cpm.2018.01.001

I will forever be grateful for his patience, kindness, and willingness to teach me his techniques.

Justin J. Fleming, DPM
University Orthopaedic Associates
2 World's Fair Drive
Somerset, NJ 08873, USA

E-mail address:
flemingjmak@gmail.com

Surgical Management Navicular and Cuboid Fractures

J. Randolph Clements, DPM[a,*], François Dijour, DPM, PGY-2[b], Wesley Leong, DPM, PGY-2[b]

KEYWORDS

- Navicular fracture • Cuboid fracture • Lateral column • Stress fracture

KEY POINTS

- It is important to recognize navicular stress fracture and organize an appropriate care plan.
- One must understand the importance of restoring the lateral column length in complex midfoot fractures.
- Understanding the diverse fixation options for navicular and cuboid fracture is critical.

ANATOMY

When navicular injuries are neglected, there are serious implications for global foot function.[1] Fusion of the talonavicular joint has been demonstrated to eliminate 91% of the original range of motion at the subtalar joint, making it the key joint of the so-called triple joint complex.[2] This complex permits three-dimensional motion between the forefoot and midfoot.

As the keystone of the medial longitudinal arch of the foot, the navicular articulates distally with the cuneiforms via three facets. These facets share a common synovial cavity. The navicular is concave on its proximal surface and articulates with the talar head. Each of the articulations are reinforced with plantar and dorsal ligaments and further stabilized by the posterior tibial tendon and plantar calcaneonavicular ligament, which insert distally and medially on the tuberosity.[3] Because of this extensive soft tissue support network, displaced navicular body fractures are typically only seen in the setting of high-energy trauma.[4]

Analysis of three-dimensional reconstructions of computed tomography (CT) images of comminuted navicular body fractures has revealed the consistent presence

Disclosure Statement: The authors have nothing to disclose.
[a] Virginia Tech-Carilion School of Medicine, 3 Riverside Circle, Roanoke, VA 24014, USA; [b] Podiatric Medical and Surgical Residency, Reconstructive Rearfoot and Ankle, Carilion Clinic, 3 Riverside Circle, Roanoke, VA 24014, USA
* Corresponding author. 3 Riverside Circle, Roanoke, VA 24016.
E-mail address: jrclements@carilionclinic.org

Clin Podiatr Med Surg 35 (2018) 145–159
https://doi.org/10.1016/j.cpm.2017.12.001
podiatric.theclinics.com

of a nondisplaced plantar lateral fragment. This piece consistently remains in contact with the cuboid bone. This fragment's relative stability has been attributed to the dense insertion of the inferior plantar calcaneonavicular ligament at this level. Reduction to this fragment has been shown to be of critical importance in obtaining the provisional stability of a heavily comminuted navicular body fracture before placing fixation.[5]

In addition to trauma, the navicular bone is also subject to repetitive injury and stress fracture. The middle one-third of the navicular body is largely avascular. Therefore, this watershed portion is most vulnerable to the long-term sequelae of stress fractures and nonunions. The extensive articular surfaces limit the available entry points by which the dorsalis pedis and medial plantar branch of the posterior tibial artery can supply the bone.[6] The combination of the previously mentioned description should remind the practitioner to maintain a high index of suspicion for navicular stress fracture (NSF) in any patient with midfoot pain.

PRESENTATION AND DIAGNOSIS

Avulsion and tuberosity fractures of the navicular are typically associated with low-energy twisting-type injuries. Fractures of the navicular body usually present following high-energy traumatic mechanisms, such as in a motor vehicle accident.[7] They often display extreme swelling and tenderness so it is imperative to rule out compartment syndrome with a detailed physical examination. Pain and swelling are localized to the dorsomedial midfoot and patients often complain of pain with push-off during gait and limited weight bearing ability.

Several different theories have been proposed for the mechanism by which navicular body injuries occur. However, most of the fractures occur secondary to abrupt axial load with a plantar flexed foot or strong dorsiflexory forces acting on the medial forefoot in the setting of hindfoot eversion.[8] CT scans are critical in the assessment of the severity of an acute navicular fracture and planning for an operative approach.[9]

NSFs are typically associated with individuals participating in rigorous sprinting or jumping activity. These account for approximately one-third of all lower extremity stress fractures. These patients most commonly present with minimal midfoot swelling and ecchymosis but complain of persistent dorsal midfoot soreness or anterior ankle pain that extends to the arch and is reproduced with explosive weight-bearing activities or direct palpation to the dorsal aspect of the talonavicular joint.[10]

MRI is considered the gold standard for early detection of stress reaction because it can identify the presence of bone marrow edema (**Fig. 1**).[11] Early recognition of such stress reactions can allow for treatment steps to be taken to prevent the development of a complete fracture. CT has been recommended as the superior modality to evaluate the navicular as it pertains to preoperative planning. CT scans provide the best visualization of the fracture line.[12] This especially holds true in the diagnosis of NSFs that have progressed to cortical disruption, for which plain radiographs have been reported to have a high incidence of false-negative results.[13] It has been the authors' experience that complete fractures are most likely to require bone grafting when compared with incomplete fractures. CT can also be used to visualize sclerosis at the fracture edges, which are more predictive of nonunion and more likely to benefit from bone grafting.

CLASSIFICATION OF INJURY

Acute navicular fractures are classified into three types: (1) avulsion, (2) tuberosity, and (3) body fractures. Acute body fractures have been further stratified into three types

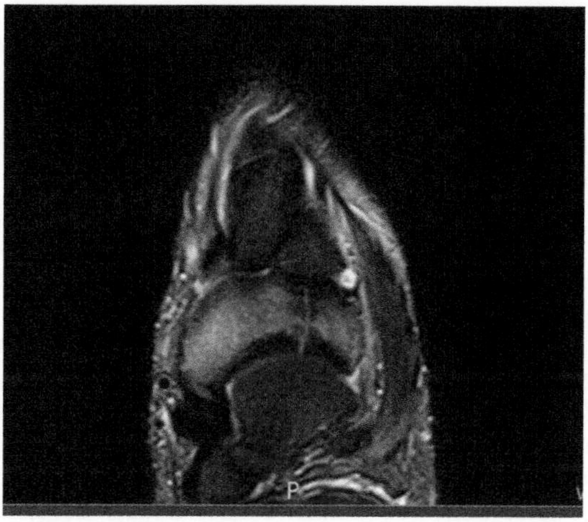

Fig. 1. Stress MRI.

based on the primary fracture line orientation and pattern of joint disruption. According to this classification by Sangeorzan and coworkers,[14] a type 1 body injury is defined as having a transverse fracture line in the coronal plane with the dorsal fragment consisting of less than 50% of the body and no disrupted alignment of the foot's medial border or forefoot angulation. A type 2 body injury is described as the most common variety and having a primary fracture line extending from dorsolateral to plantar-medial with concomitant medial displacement of the forefoot. There is often associated rupture of the dorsal talonavicular ligament. A type 3 body injury has a comminuted fracture in the sagittal plane of the navicular body with concomitant lateral displacement of the forefoot medial disruption at the naviculocuneiform joint. These injuries are often associated with extensive damage to the calcaneocuboid joint.[4]

NSFs have been organized into a classification system by Saxena and Fullem[12] who correlated NSF healing times with the degree of severity as observed on coronal views of CT imaging. Type 1 NSFs are described as having a dorsal cortical interruption without intrabody extension. In type 2 NSFs the fracture line is seen extending into the navicular body itself, whereas to be considered a type 3 NSF, there must be complete propagation of the fracture line into a second cortex (medial, lateral, or plantar). A signal change noted on MRI without concomitant CT signs of a cortical break was later classified as a type 0.5 NSF.

TREATMENT

Avulsion fractures are typically managed nonoperatively in a supportive shoe, cast boot, or short leg walking cast. It is possible to manage simple nondisplaced body fractures with immobilization and protected weightbearing in a short leg cast as long as serial radiographs are assessed monthly for any interval displacement that requires surgical intervention.

Indications for surgical repair of navicular body fractures include medial column shortening greater than 2 mm, displacement of the joint or incongruity of greater than 1 mm, concomitant lateral column damage, gross instability, compartment syndrome, or irreducible dislocation. The primary goals for open reduction and internal fixation include anatomic restoration of the talonavicular joint and medial column length using rigid fixation that could allow for early range of motion.[15] To prevent recurrent talonavicular subluxation, at least 60% of the navicular's proximal articular surface needs to be restored.[8] Severely comminuted navicular body fractures with extensive destruction of the articular surfaces may not be amenable to open reduction internal fixation because of the pivotal role its articulations play in global foot function. These cases may require primary medial column arthrodesis, spanning external fixation or temporary medial column bridge plating.[16]

With regards to the management of stress fractures, some studies have reported that conservative treatment provides the most successful outcomes regardless of fracture pattern. However, this remains a topic of considerable debate and Saxena and colleagues[13] proposed an algorithm based on his classification system in which type 0.5 and type 1 NSFs were treated with short leg casts and immobilization. Patients with type 2 and 3 NSFs are urged to strongly consider primary surgical fixation to lower the risk of refracture or malunion. Unfortunately, no high-level studies exist at this time that draw conclusions regarding the optimum treatment to achieve the earliest return to activity and lower incidence of refracture. In the authors' experience, patients who are athletes undergoing either conservative or surgical management of their stress fracture can expect to lose at least one season of their sport before making a full return to normal activity.

OPERATIVE TECHNIQUE GUIDE

Stress Fractures

After appropriate care of the soft tissues and higher priority injuries, the patient is positioned supine on the operating table with a thigh tourniquet. A dorsomedial approach to the foot is performed with a 4-cm incision starting proximally at the ankle joint and medial to the tibialis anterior tendon. The incision is extended laterally over the tibialis anterior insertion at the medial cuneiform and carried distally to the midportion of the dorsomedial first metatarsal. During dissection through the subcutaneous tissues, ligation and coagulation of the venous branches of the saphenous vein is performed while care is taken to preserve the branches of the saphenous and superficial peroneal nerves.

The tibialis anterior and extensor hallucis longus tendons are identified and protected throughout the procedure using blunt retraction. Dissection is continued onto the dorsal aspect of the fractured tarsal navicular where the articular surfaces are visualized and the fracture site identified once all fibrous tissue is excised. All sclerotic bone is removed with a rongeur. This step is essential to preventing a nonunion, so particular care should be taken during this step. A drill bit may be used to drill medially and laterally through the fracture site to further stimulate local blood flow. The tourniquet should be released at this time to visualize adequate sclerotic bone removal by observing return of blood to the fracture site.

Our team typically uses autologous bone graft for this fracture when CT suggests the fracture is complete and/or has sclerotic lines. Typically this low autograft volume can be harvested from the calcaneus. This is done through a small stab incision made in the posterior lateral third aspect of the calcaneus. Blunt dissection is carried down to the calcaneus bone and a small reamer used to obtain the autograft after making two passes, each of which are roughly 15 mm deep. The harvest site can be backfilled with allograft bone chips.

The freshly harvested autograft is packed into the fracture site with a bone tamp. A clamp is used to oppose the fracture ends and two opposing parallel screws of 3.5 mm or 4 mm diameter are placed from the medial and lateral sides of the navicular. The first screw can be positioned superiorly and proximally relative to the second screw. Appropriate positioning is confirmed using fluoroscopy. Care is taken to avoid screw impingement on the posterior tibial tendon or into the talonavicular or cuneonavicular joint (**Fig. 2**).

The postoperative course consists of nonweightbearing for 2 weeks in a posterior splint, followed by 6 to 8 more weeks of nonweightbearing in a controlled ankle motion boot. Our practice allows the patient to remove the controlled ankle motion boot for nonweightbearing range of motion exercises. Protected weightbearing as tolerated is started at 8 to 12 weeks. Return to full unprotected weight bearing is not allowed until healing is confirmed by CT scan, the first of which is usually obtained at 10 to 12 weeks postoperatively. In the case of athletes, return to play is usually delayed by at least 6 months, depending on the recovery progress and demands of the particular sport.

Plate Fixation of Acute Navicular Body Fractures

After appropriate care of the soft tissues and higher priority injuries, the patient is positioned supine on the operating table with a thigh tourniquet. Most navicular fractures are accessed with a dorsomedial incision centered over the talonavicular joint. Minor adjustments are made to the incision depending on the site of the primary fracture. This is determined by careful scrutiny of the preoperative radiographs and CT scans. The standard dorsomedial incision starting proximally at the ankle joint and medial to the tibialis anterior tendon is extended laterally over the tibialis anterior insertion at the medial cuneiform and carried distally over the navicular body as necessary to expose the fracture site. During dissection through the subcutaneous tissues, ligation and coagulation of the venous branches of the saphenous vein is performed while care is taken to preserve the branches of the saphenous and superficial peroneal nerves (**Figs. 3–5**).

Fractures that are centered over the lateral aspect of navicular are accessed between the extensor hallucis longus and extensor digitorum longus tendons. Alternatively, fractures that are more centrally located in the body of the navicular are accessed in the interval between extensor hallucis longus and tibialis anterior tendons. The deep peroneal nerve and dorsalis pedis artery are mobilized and retracted laterally together with the extensor digitorum longus tendon. Full exposure of the spherical joint surfaces is obtained by using a mini distractor placed between the talar neck and medial cuneiform. These distraction devices can also be used to help restore the length of the medial column and provides improved visualization of the articular

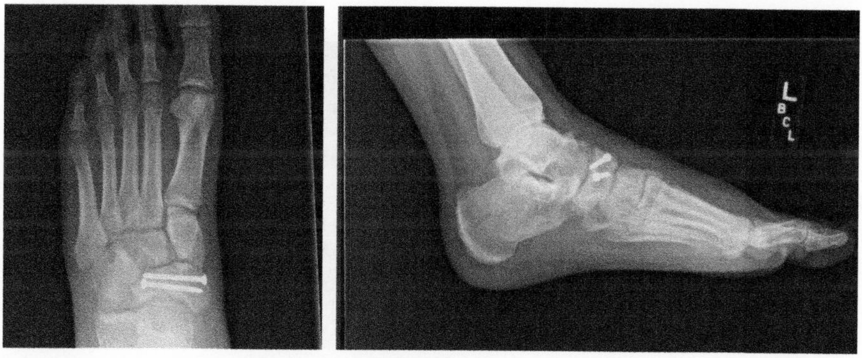

Fig. 2. Open reduction internal fixation later stress.

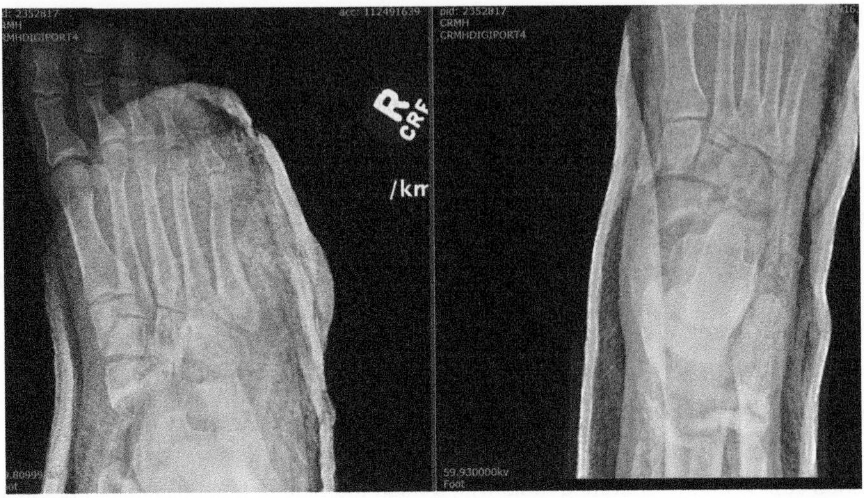

Fig. 3. Navicular 1.

reduction. If possible, the articular capsule should be opened on the side of the talus so as to preserve as much of the navicular vascularization as possible.

Once the hematoma and fibrous debris is appropriately excised and irrigated from the fracture site, the main fragments are identified and carefully mobilized. The surgeon should seek to identify the location of the lateral plantar fragment. Again, this fragment has been demonstrated to be consistently nondisplaced in comminuted navicular body fractures. Initial stability is obtained through the use of pointed reduction forceps to compress fragments against the lateral plantar fragment in a dorsolateral position. Temporary fixation with K-wires using a stepwise approach is performed as needed. Once again, the authors emphasize the importance of starting with the more constant plantar fragments and then progressing from a lateral to medial direction.

Autologous bone graft is used to fill any central compression defects. After a reduction forceps is used to clamp the navicular tuberosity fragment to the reconstructed navicular body, compression screws are placed through a smaller incision to achieve final fixation. Simple fracture patterns are addressed with 2.7- and 3.5-mm screws. The more complex or comminuted fractures are more amenable to anatomically shaped dorsal locking plates. To preserve the vascularity to the navicular, the plate

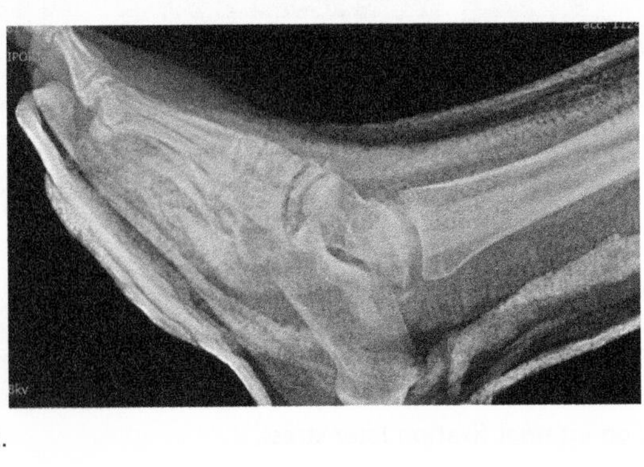

Fig. 4. Navicular 2.

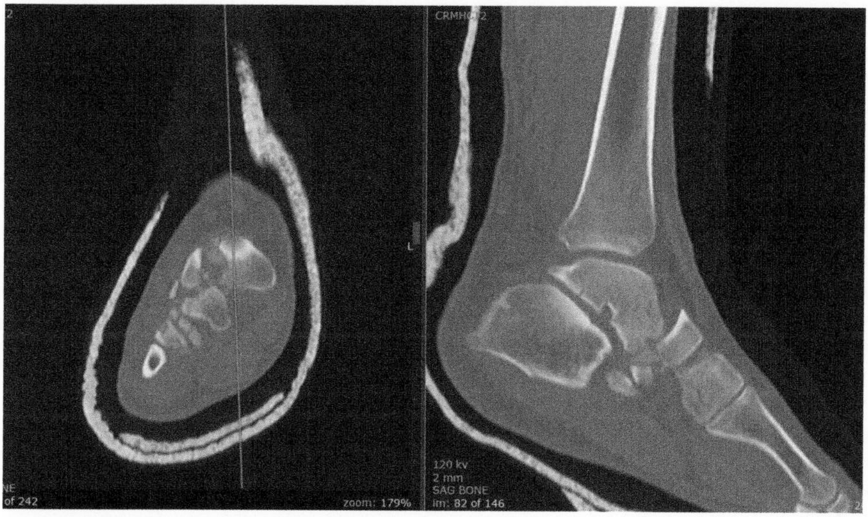

Fig. 5. Navicular 3.

must be slipped under the soft tissues without releasing the dorsal periosteum if possible.[5] The plate must be cut to the appropriate length and formed so that the angle of the screws faces away from the adjacent articular surface.

Following confirmation of the proper hardware placement under fluoroscopy, multiple locking screws are placed with care being taken to avoid entering the talonavicular or naviculocuneiform joints. Screws closest to the talonavicular joint should be directed at a slightly distal angle so as to avoid penetrating the extremely concave talonavicular joint. The fluoroscopy images should be multiplanar to ensure there is no transarticular hardware placement. After repair of the joint capsules and extensor retinaculum, a layered wound closure is performed. The postoperative course consists of splint and cast immobilization with progressive weightbearing initiated after 8 to 12 weeks (**Fig. 6**).

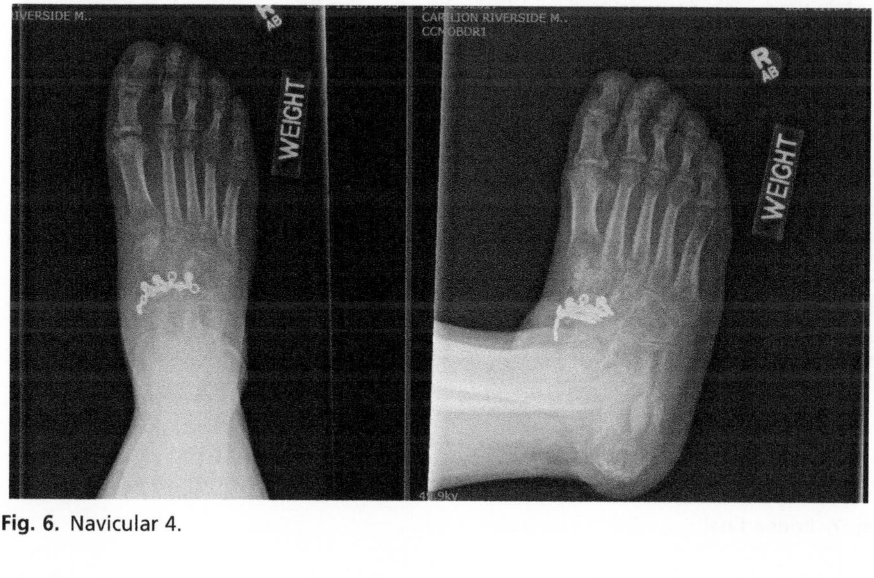

Fig. 6. Navicular 4.

Temporary Medial Bridge Plating of Heavily Comminuted Navicular Body Fractures

The standard dorsomedial incision is initiated as previously described and extended distally to reveal the midportion of the dorsomedial first metatarsal. Dissection to the navicular bone proceeds as previously described but the extensor retinaculum needs to be transected to allow for bridge plating onto the talar neck.

After provisional stabilization of the large bony fragments is achieved with K-wires, a temporary two-point external fixator is used to reconstitute the alignment and length of the medial column by placing it between the distal aspect of the first metatarsal and the calcaneus. An 8- to 10-hole 2.7-mm reconstruction plate is then slid underneath the tibialis anterior tendon and placed over the medial aspect of the medial column of the foot. Special care should be taken to avoid disrupting tibialis anterior tendon or its insertion. The plate is secured to the talar neck by two 2.7-mm screws into the talar neck and two more into the first metatarsal (**Fig. 7**).

An additional screw can be placed through the plate into the medial cuneiform extending into the remaining cuneiforms while another screw is placed through the medial cuneiform into the second and third metatarsal bases. After repair of the joint capsules and extensor retinaculum, a layered wound closure is performed.

After a 12-week postoperative period of nonweightbearing, a staged removal of the medial column bridge plate is planned for 3 months postoperatively. The plate is initially shortened by selectively removing the segment overlying the talonavicular joint and thereby allowing for continued stabilization of the midfoot while full weightbearing is initiated and advanced according to clinical and radiographic assessment.[17–19]

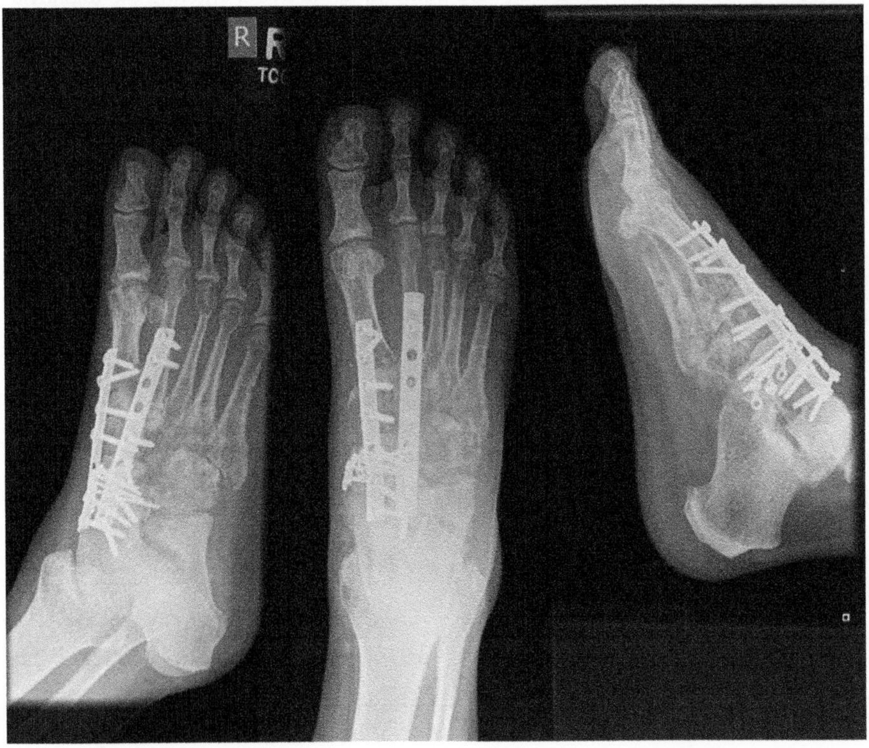

Fig. 7. Bridee final.

CUBOID FRACTURE

Abstract

Cuboid fractures are not uncommonly associated with concurrent fractures or injuries of the midfoot or medial column. The mechanism of injury resulting in a cuboid fracture may be a direct impact to the cuboid or from indirect force acting on the cuboid from the foot and ankle. Typically the mechanism in an indirect injury is a rotational force in a plantarflexed position and abduction, causing the cuboid to get crushed between its adjacent articulations with the calcaneus and metatarsals.[20] A cuboid crush injury (also known as a "nutcracker" injury) may be subtle on plain film radiographs; however, it is important to recognize and treat appropriately because of the possibility of significantly compromised foot biomechanics. Failure to address a cuboid crush injury may result in pes planus deformity and late instability.

Anatomy

The main function of the cuboid bone is to maintain the length of the lateral column while providing critical articulation points for most of the lateral column. The fourth and fifth tarsometatarsal articulations between the cuboid and metatarsals provide as much as three times the motion as compared with the first through third tarsometatarsal articulations.[21,22] The mobility of the lateral column is an important contributor to the foot's ability to adapt to uneven terrain.[23,24] Compromise of the motion of these joints has significant ramifications on the biomechanics of the foot.

Presentation and Diagnosis

Patients presenting with lateral foot pain and multiple midfoot injuries including high-energy Lisfranc injuries should be closely evaluated for a concurrent lateral column insult and concurrent cuboid injury. Swelling, deformity, ecchymosis, or fracture blisters may be seen with a cuboid fracture. Typically there is tenderness to direct palpation of the cuboid.

Generally plain film radiographs with anteroposterior, lateral, and oblique views are adequate in visualizing a cuboid fracture. The medial oblique view is important in assessing the cuboid because this view shows the cuboid and its articulations free of superimposition with open and equal cuboid joint spaces. Once the cuboid fracture diagnosis is made, a CT scan is useful to fully appreciate the nature of the fracture and in selecting the appropriate treatment. Contralateral films may be useful for comparison in subtle injuries and for surgical planning (**Figs. 8–10**).

There is no universally used classification system for cuboid fractures; however, cuboid fractures can largely be grouped into extra-articular/intra-articular, displaced/nondisplaced, avulsion, or crush type injury.

Treatment

Nonoperative management of cuboid fractures is appropriate in the setting of an avulsion or nondisplaced fracture particularly without any impaction or compromise of lateral column length. Nondisplaced fractures should be kept nonweightbearing in a short leg cast for 6 to 8 weeks, at which time weightbearing radiographs are obtained to evaluate fracture healing and cuboid instability sequelae. Cuboid avulsion fractures may be managed with immediate protected weightbearing as tolerated in a fracture boot for 4 to 6 weeks.

Operative management of cuboid fractures is indicated when an articular step-off greater than 2 mm exists or if there is any shortening of the lateral column.[22] Historically, multiple options for fixation have been described including open reduction and

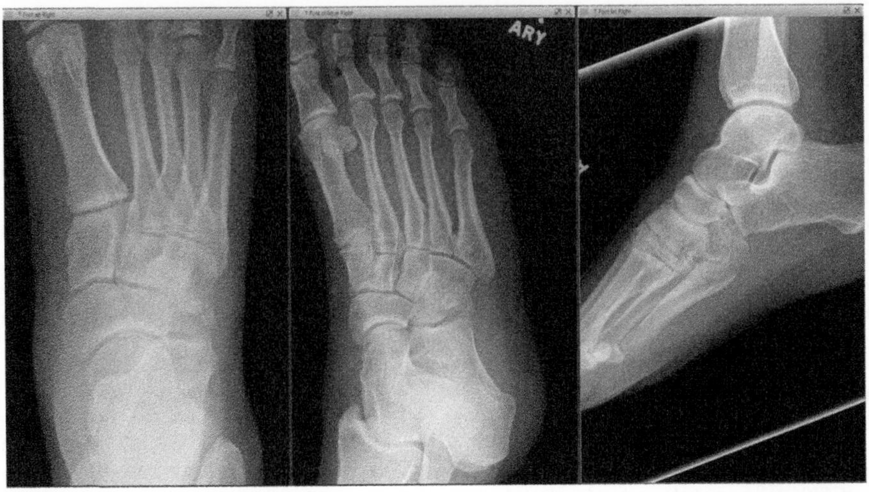

Fig. 8. Cuboid plate A.

internal fixation using a locking anatomic plate or open reduction and stabilization with external fixation. In a severe crush injury with extensive comminution, spanning external fixation is recommended to restore lateral column length; an alternative and albeit controversial management is primary arthrodesis. The authors advise against this in normally sensate patients because of the significant loss in lateral column motion. In the setting of concurrent medial column, and/or midtarsal injury, it is critical to first restore lateral column length and to adequately stabilize the lateral column. Once the lateral column length has been restored and stabilized, the medial column should return to a gross anatomic alignment. This allows for complete anatomic reduction with subsequent definitive fixation. In cases with lateral column shortening secondary to cuboid impaction when the length cannot be restored with closed reduction and external fixator application, an open procedure needs to be performed. These cases require substantial use of bone grafting to fill the cancellous void.[20] An open procedure likely needs to be used in the case of a malunion secondary to a missed crushed injury (**Fig. 11**).[25]

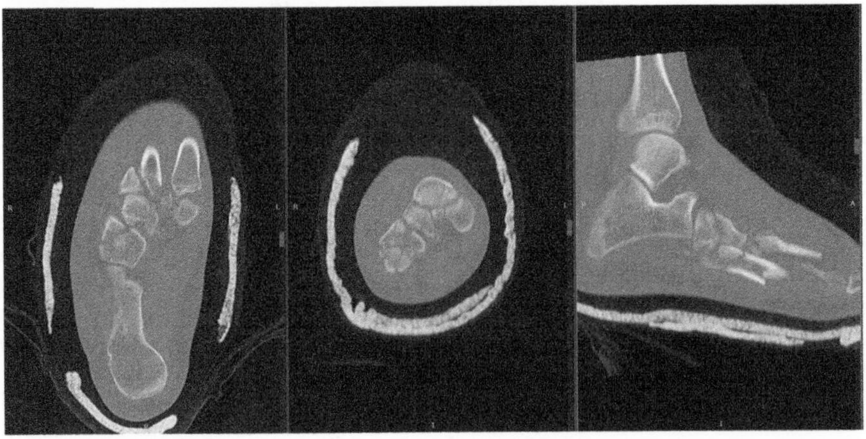
Fig. 9. Cuboid rail B.

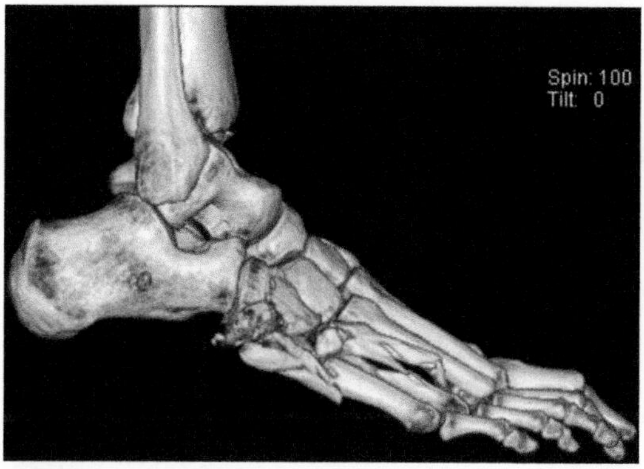

Fig. 10. Cuboid rail C.

OPERATIVE TECHNIQUE

Cuboid Intra-Articular Fracture

The patient is placed supine on the operating room table with an ipsilateral hip bump. The lower extremity is exsanguinated and a thigh tourniquet is inflated. A 6-cm longitudinal incision is made directly over the cuboid at the dorsolateral foot. Dissection is carried deep to the extensor digitorum brevis and then the muscle belly is reflected off the periosteum and retracted dorsally. The cuboid is visualized and the calcaneocuboid and tarsometatarsal joints are inspected. A Freer elevator is used to mobilize the fracture and a small tenaculum is used to reduce the fracture. The cuboid articulations are visualized under fluoroscopy to confirm anatomic reduction and joint congruity. An anatomic plate is then secured to the cuboid using nonlocking and locking screws (**Fig. 12**).

Cuboid Crush Injury

The first line of treatment is application of a monorail adjustable (distraction) external fixator laterally in the acute setting and closed reduction of the cuboid. The pins are placed into the fifth metatarsal diaphysis distally and into the calcaneus proximally.

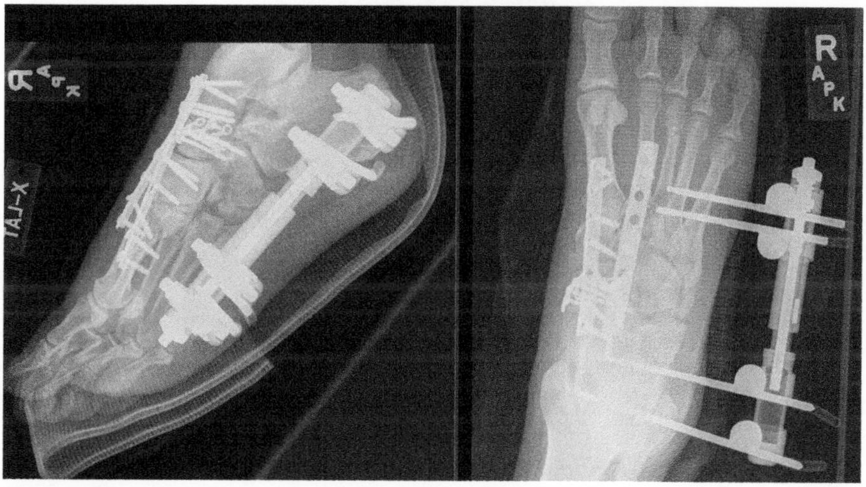

Fig. 11. Bridge 2.

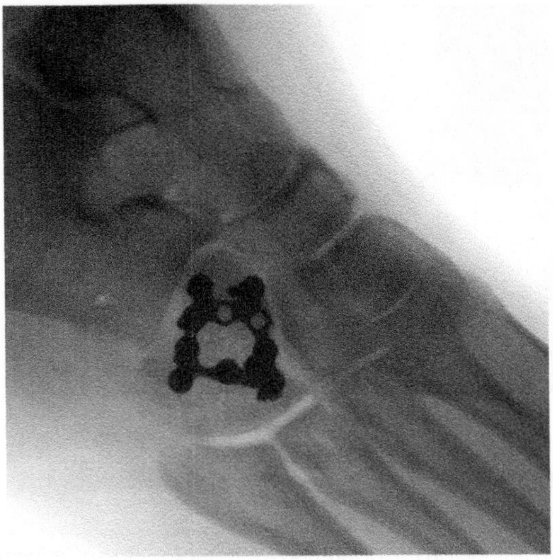

Fig. 12. Cuboid plate D.

The soft tissue envelope is likely not amenable to open treatment because of swelling. The goals of treatment are restoration of lateral column length and prevention of soft tissue contracture. The patient may have a concurrent medial column injury; this may be addressed in the future once soft tissue allows. If lateral column length remains short after external fixation, then it is recommended to proceed with open treatment once the soft tissue envelope resuscitates. This may be seen in subacute cases where the impaction injury was missed and bone healing has begun.

Patient positioning and dissection is the same as the nonimpacted cuboid injury. Once the cuboid is fully exposed, attention is now shifted away from the cuboid and the entire foot is analyzed under direct fluoroscopy. The lateral column is

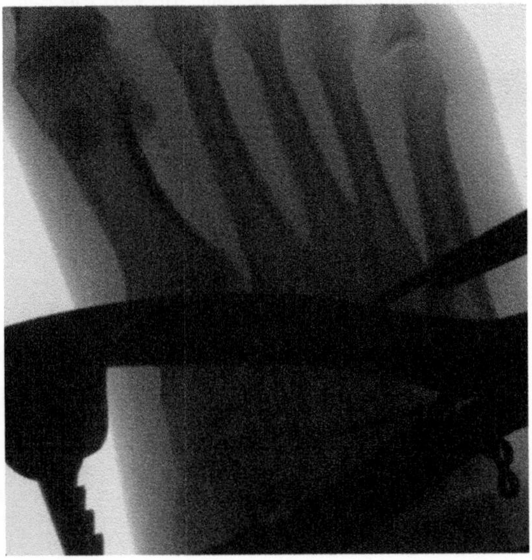

Fig. 13. Cuboid plate B.

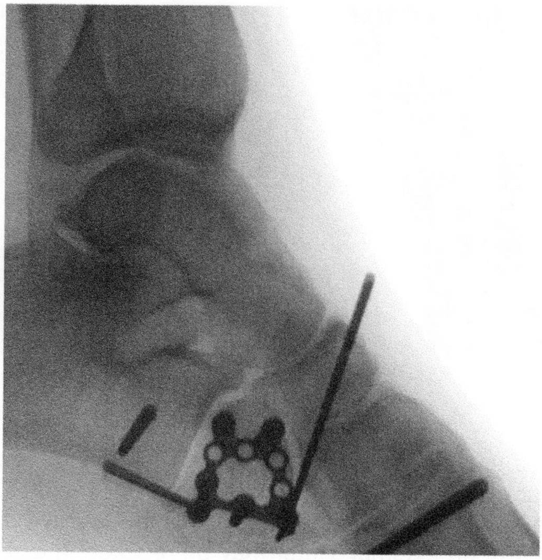

Fig. 14. Cuboid plate C.

inspected and the amount of shortening is noted and the degree of abduction is appreciated medially via talar head uncoverage at the talonavicular joint. Attention is then redirected to the cuboid where the dorsolateral cortex of the cuboid is lifted with a Freer in an eggshell fashion. The critical portion of the case is now fully disimpacting the cuboid and restoring anatomic length of the lateral column. This author uses a Hintermann distractor with the pins placed within the proximal and distal portions of the cuboid (**Figs. 13** and **14**). Gentle distraction pressure is applied. The impacted cancellous bone may require mobilization with a Cobb elevator or blunt instrument, particularly if boney callus has formed preventing distraction. Care is taken not to perforate the bone into the joint space. Gentle distraction is continued segmentally as the cancellous bone of the cuboid is disimpacted as needed. The lateral

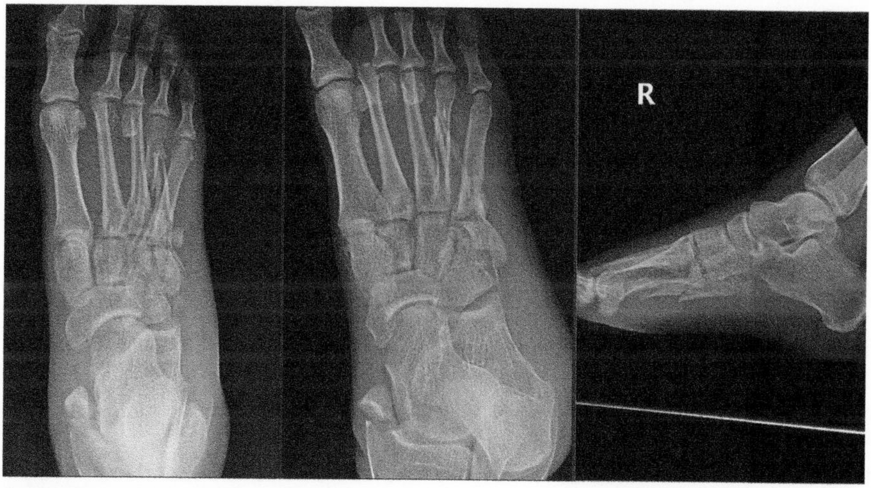

Fig. 15. Cuboid rail A.

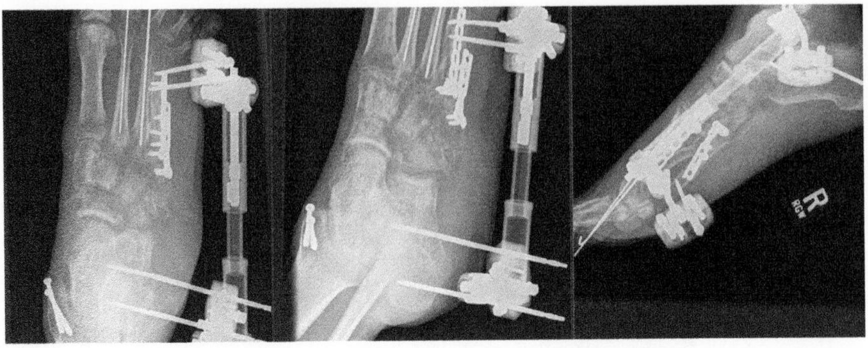

Fig. 16. Cuboid rail D.

column is inspected under fluoroscopy for restoration of length and observation of increased talar head coverage. Once the cuboid length is restored, the void is filled with cancellous bone chips. An anatomic plate is placed over the cuboid to maintain length. The addition of an external fixator may be required in cases with extensive comminution not amenable to plate fixation. The extensor digitorum brevis muscle belly is repaired back to the periosteum and the wound is closed in a layered fashion. Once the lateral column length is restored, the remainder of the midfoot procedures may be performed. The postoperative course includes nonweightbearing for 8 to 12 weeks followed by 4 weeks of protected weightbearing in a fracture boot (**Figs. 15** and **16**).

REFERENCES

1. Rosenbaum AJ, Uhl R, DiPreta J. Acute fractures of the tarsal navicular. Orthopedics 2014;37(8):541–6.
2. Astion DJ, Deland JT, Otis JC, et al. Motion of the hindfoot after simulated arthrodesis. J Bone Joint Surg Am 1997;79:241–6.
3. Sarrafian SK, Kekilian AS. Functional Anatomy of the Foot and Ankle. In: Sarrafian SK, Kekilian AS, editors. Sarrafian's anatomy of the foot and ankle, Descriptive, Topographic, Functional. 3rd edition. Philadelphia: Wolters Kluwer, Lippincott Williams & Wilkins; 2011.
4. Rammelt S, Schepers T. Chopart injuries: when to fix and when to fuse? Foot Ankle Clin N Am 2017;22:163–80.
5. Cronier P, Frin JM, Steiger V, et al. Internal fixation of complex fractures of the tarsal navicular with locking plates. A report of 10 cases. Orthop Traumatol Surg Res 2013;99S:S241–9.
6. Golano P, Farinas O, Saenz I. The anatomy of the navicular and periarticular structures. Foot Ankle Clin 2004;9:1–23.
7. Eichenholtz SN, Levine DB. Fractures of the tarsal navicular bone. Clin Orthop Relat Res 1964;34:142–57.
8. Main BJ, Jowett RL. Injuries of the midtarsal joint. J Bone Joint Surg Br 1975;57:89–97.
9. Rammelt S, Grass R, Zwipp H. Nutcracker fractures of the navicular and cuboid. Ther Umsch 2004;61:451–7.
10. Jones MH, Amendola AS. Navicular stress fractures. Clin Sports Med 2006;25:151–8.

11. Boden BP, Osbahr DC. High-risk stress fractures: evaluation and treatment. J Am Acad Orthop Surg 2000;8(6):344–53.
12. Saxena A, Fullem B. A unique procedure for treatment of 22 navicular stress fractures: a new proposed radiographic classification system. J Foot Ankle Surg 2000;39:96–103.
13. Saxena A, Beham S, Valerio D, et al. Navicular stress fracture outcomes in athletes: analysis of 62 injuries. J Foot Ankle Surg 2017;56:943–8.
14. Sangeorzan BJ, Benirschke SK, Mosca V, et al. Displaced intra-articular fractures of the tarsal navicular. J Bone Joint Surg Am 1989;71(10):1504–10.
15. Banerjee R, Nickisch F, Easley M, et al. Foot injuries. In: Browner B, Jupiter J, Levine A, et al, editors. Skeletal trauma. Philadelphia: WB Saunders; 2008. p. 2671–2.
16. Rammelt S. Chopart and Lisfranc joint injuries. In: Bentley G, editor. European surgical orthopaedics and traumatology. The EFORT textbook. Berlin: Springer; 2014. p. 3835–57.
17. Apostle KL, Younger ASE. Technique tip: open reduction internal fixation of comminuted fractures of the navicular with bridge plating to the medial and middle cuneiforms. Foot Ankle Int 2008;29(7):739–41.
18. Bayley E, Duncan N, Taylor A. The use of locking plates in complex midfoot fractures. Ann R Coll Surg Engl 2012;94:593–6.
19. Schildhauer TA, Nork SE, Sangeorzan BJ. Temporary bridge plating of the medial column in severe midfoot injuries. J Orthop Trauma 2003;17(7):513–20.
20. Mihalich RM, Early JS. Management of cuboid crush injuries. Foot Ankle Clin 2006;11:121–6.
21. Ouzounian TJ, Shereff MJ. In vitro determination of midfoot motion. Foot Ankle 1989;10:140–6.
22. Yu X, Pang QJ, Yu GR. The injuries to the fourth and fifth tarsometatarsal joints: A review of the surgical management by internal fixation, arthrodesis and arthroplasty. Pak J Med Sci 2013;29(2):687–92.
23. Patel A, Rao S, Nawoczenski D, et al. Midfoot arthritis. J Am Acad Orthop Surg 2010;18:417–25.
24. Rockwood CA Jr, Green DP, Bucholz RW. Rockwood and green's fractures in adults.. In: Bucholz RW, Heckman JD, Court-Brown CM, editors. Fractures in adults. 6th edition. Philadelphia: Lippincott Williams & Wilkins; 2006.
25. Yu G, Yu T, Yang Y, et al. Old nutcracker fracture of cuboid. Indian J Orthop 2013;47(3):310–2.

Management of Talar Fractures

Kwasi Y. Kwaadu, DPM

KEYWORDS

• Avascular necrosis • Malunion • Post-traumatic osteoarthritis • Talar fracture • Talus

KEY POINTS

- Talar fractures are life-changing events. As such, their outcomes should realistically be tempered.
- Along with preoperative advanced imaging, the threshold for operative and accurate anatomic reduction should be low.
- Dual incisional approaches and malleolar osteotomies increase visualization to help facilitate accurate and anatomic reduction.
- Avoiding extensive subperiosteal dissection minimizes disruption of the already acutely traumatized tenuous perfusion.
- Although avascular necrosis can prove a devastating sequelae of this injury, it occurs far less frequently that posttraumatic osteoarthritis many times warranting secondary operations.

INTRODUCTION

The talus has a unique architecture with varying fracture presentation from simple avulsions about the head and neck secondary to inversion ankle sprains, and fractures of the lateral process and posterior tubercles from sudden, unplanned, and sometimes atypical mechanisms and motion. Although these former injuries are at times operative, they have not historically been associated with the sequelae and complications seen with complete fractures of the neck and intra-articular fractures of the wholly articular body/trochlear (**Fig. 1**).[1] These latter injuries have historically proven difficult to manage for even highly trained foot and ankle traumatologists.[1–5] The complex anatomy of the talus contributes to the difficulty in visualization, reduction, and the real estate available for fixation (**Fig. 2**).

Multiple classification systems have been provided in the past but the Hawkins classification system described in 1970 has continued to be relied on to offer

Disclosure: The author has nothing to disclose.
Department of Surgery, Temple University School of Podiatric Medicine, 148 North 8th Street, Philadelphia, PA 19107, USA
E-mail address: kwasi.kwaadu@temple.edu

Clin Podiatr Med Surg 35 (2018) 161–173
https://doi.org/10.1016/j.cpm.2017.12.007
podiatric.theclinics.com

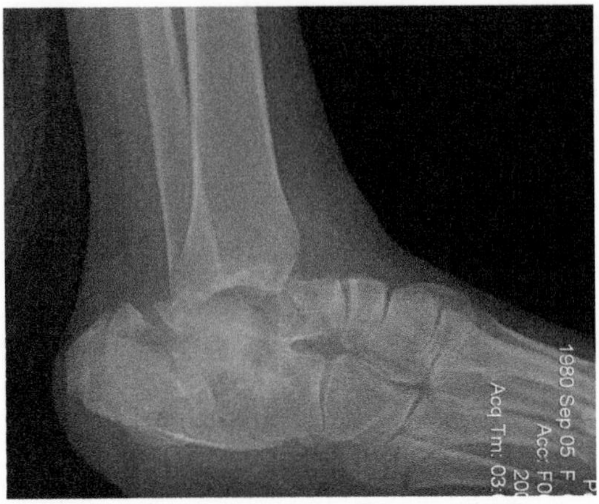

Fig. 1. Severe fracture of the talar trochlear with associated calcaneal fracture. (*Courtesy of* Justin J. Fleming, DPM, American College of Foot and Ankle Surgeons, Philadelphia, PA.)

a foundational understanding of these injuries, correlating progressive displacement and articular dislocation with prognosis.[5–7] This has led to subsequent research that has further increased the understanding of these injuries, providing more contemporary clinical pictures of associated sequelae.[8] Historical recommendations emphasized early open reduction, correlating this with a reduced incidence of avascular necrosis and collapse as a consequence of the timelier restoration of the surrounding perfusion (**Fig. 3**).[9–14] However, these high-energy injuries many times traumatize the surrounding soft tissues, making early open reduction difficult (**Fig. 4**). Furthermore, Vallier and colleagues[15] demonstrated no clear correlation with operative timing with the incidence of avascular necrosis. Finally, and even in the presence of avascular necrosis, collapse is not uniformly imminent.[9–14,16]

Sneppen and coworkers[17] proposed a classification system for fractures of the body. The classification system is descriptive, but unlike the Hawkins classification, has provided no discrete and clear correlation with prognosis. Unlike fractures of

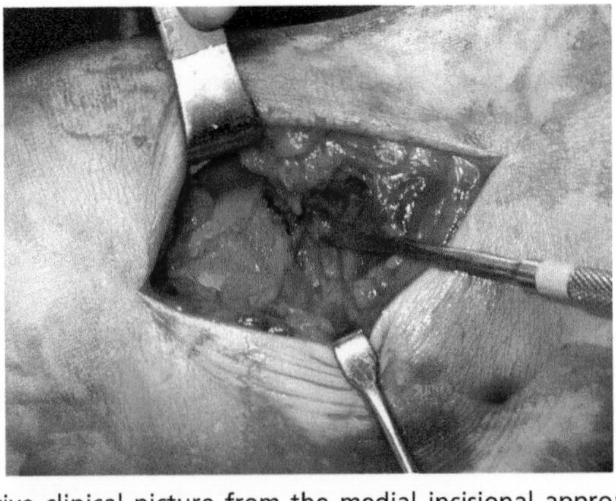

Fig. 2. Intraoperative clinical picture from the medial incisional approach demonstrating limited area for plate fixation. (*Courtesy of* Justin J. Fleming, DPM, American College of Foot and Ankle Surgeons, Philadelphia, PA.)

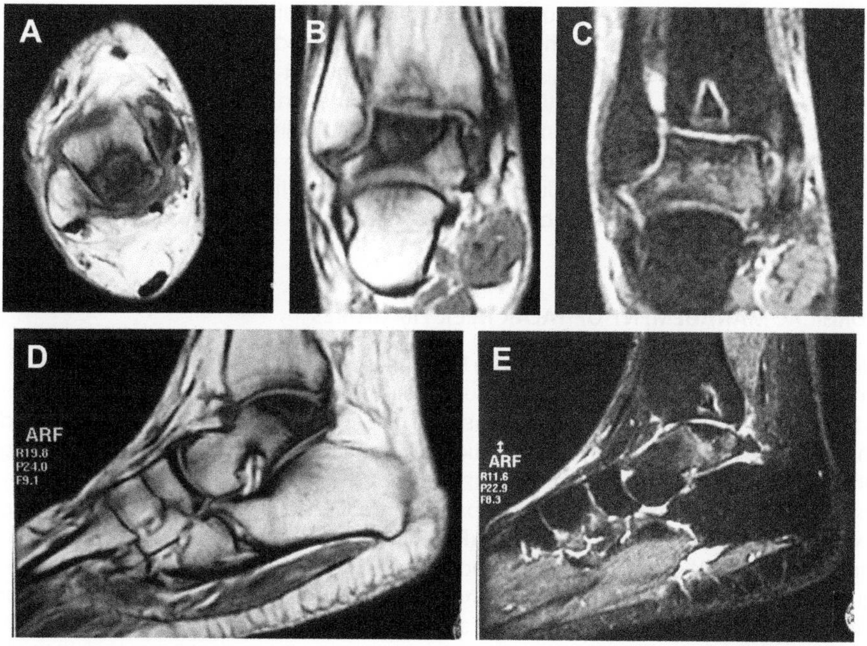

Fig. 3. Multiple MRIs of an individual with avascular necrosis of the talus, potential sequelae of talar neck fractures. (*A*) T1 axial MRI with hypointensity along the posterolateral talar dome demonstrating avascular necrosis. (*B*) T1 coronal MRI with hypointensity along the posterolateral talar dome demonstrating avascular necrosis. Along the distal tibia, there is a hypointense area consistent with a bone infarct. (*C*) T2 short tau inversion recovery coronal MRI of the same study with increased inflammation diffusely within the talar body. There is a bone infarct along the distal tibia with a surrounding rim of inflammatory tissue. (*D*) T1 sagittal MRI with hypointensity along the posterior talar dome demonstrating avascular necrosis. (*E*) T2 short tau inversion recovery MRI with hyperintensity along the posterior talar dome demonstrating avascular necrosis. (*Courtesy of* Justin J. Fleming, DPM, American College of Foot and Ankle Surgeons, Philadelphia, PA.)

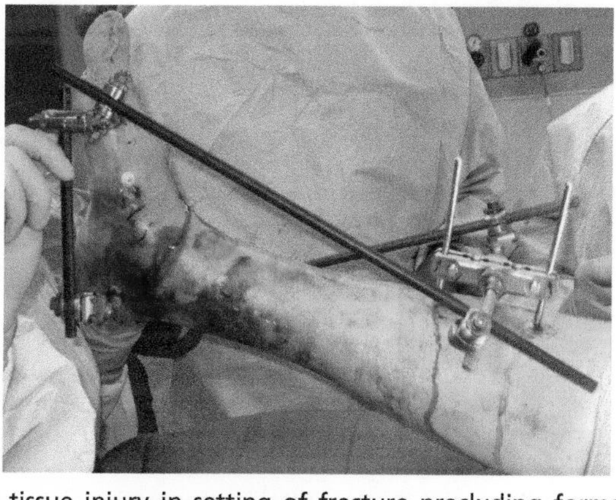

Fig. 4. Severe soft tissue injury in setting of fracture precluding formal open reduction. There is an applied external fixator. *Courtesy* of Justin J. Fleming, DPM, American College of Foot and Ankle Surgeons, Philadelphia, PA.

the neck that occur as a consequence of cantilever bending of the talar neck on the locked hindfoot, fractures of the body are likely secondary to high-energy forces that axially trap the talar body, subsequently crushing it between the talar plafond and the calcaneus.[18] Wholly articular and well secured in the ankle mortise, access for accurate anatomic reduction and safe locations for internal fixation delivery are challenging. Fractures/dislocations of the talar body are not subtle injuries that are readily missed (**Fig. 5**).[19] Standard anteroposterior, mortise, and lateral projections of ankle radiographs are helpful but advanced imaging is a necessity for accurate fracture reduction planning.

SURGICAL MANAGEMENT OF TALAR NECK FRACTURES

Hawkins type I fractures of the neck are those through and through fractures with minimal displacement. These fracture are successfully treated with cast immobilization for 6 to 8 weeks.[20] However, even in the absence of displacement, internal fixation placed through small incisions provides additional internal stabilization, giving the treating physician and patient the confidence to begin early range of motion physical therapy exercises, even during the nonweightbearing recovery phase, limiting stiffness and expediting an earlier return to function (**Fig. 6**).[21] This early mobilization can also provide some protection against deep venous thrombus formation as a potential consequence of complete cast immobilization that could further increase morbidity. Even in the absence of obvious displacement, subtle varus malalignment may be imperceptible radiographically as a consequence of the complex anatomy of the talus and hindfoot osseous structures, making preoperative computed tomography a necessity.[22] Some simple type I fractures are difficult to appreciate radiographically and in the absence of advanced imaging, the injury could be missed entirely and potentially mistreated.

Hawkins II fractures with subtalar joint displacement and III fractures with displacement of both the subtalar and ankle joints require immediate closed reduction, with the ankle splinted in plantarflexion to prevent redisplacement (**Fig. 7**). Hawkins III fractures that fail closed reduction require operative reduction (**Fig. 8**). Rush and Hamilton[21]

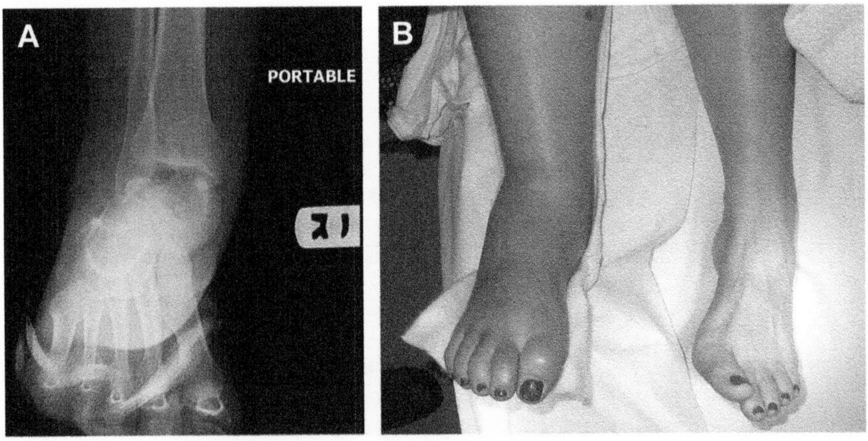

Fig. 5. Anteroposterior radiograph (*A*) and clinical intraoperative picture of a grade III talar fracture (*B*). (*Courtesy of* Justin J. Fleming, DPM, American College of Foot and Ankle Surgeons, Philadelphia, PA.)

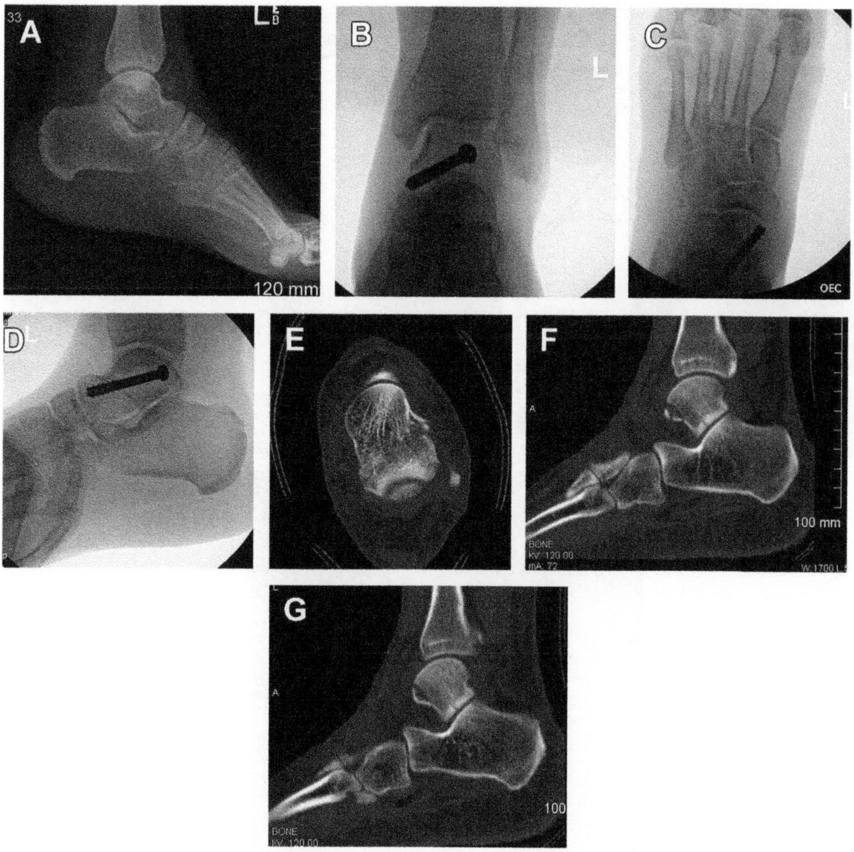

Fig. 6. (*A–G*) Preoperative axial and sagittal computed tomographic images of a minimally displaced talar along with the intraoperative fluoroscopic film following open reduction and internal fixation with an anterograde place cannulated screw. (*Courtesy of* Justin J. Fleming, DPM, American College of Foot and Ankle Surgeons, Philadelphia, PA.)

recommended initial reduction facilitated with external fixation in lieu of formal open reduction.

Dual anteromedial and anterolateral approaches are generally recommended to reduce varus malalignment in the frontal plane that may occur with the use of an isolated anteromedial incisional approach as a consequence of missed comminution and generally reduced visualization.[23–28] The concern for the additional soft tissue dissection with the dual approach has been theorized to further compromise vascular supply. However, in the absence of extensive subperiosteal stripping, it has not been substantiated to further disrupt vascular supply significantly enough to increase risk of avascular necrosis.[10–15,29] The dual incisions are centered along the lateral radiographic longitudinal bisection of the talar neck (see **Fig. 8**). The lateral incision courses adjacent the lateral branch of the intermediate dorsocutaneous nerve and lateral to the lateral-most slip of the extensor digitorum longus tendon. The medial incision runs medially and inferiorly to the tibialis anterior tendon and superior to the posterior tibial tendon immediately adjacent to the course of the medial marginal vein. These incisions allow for excellent visualization of the neck fracture and the subtalar joint where

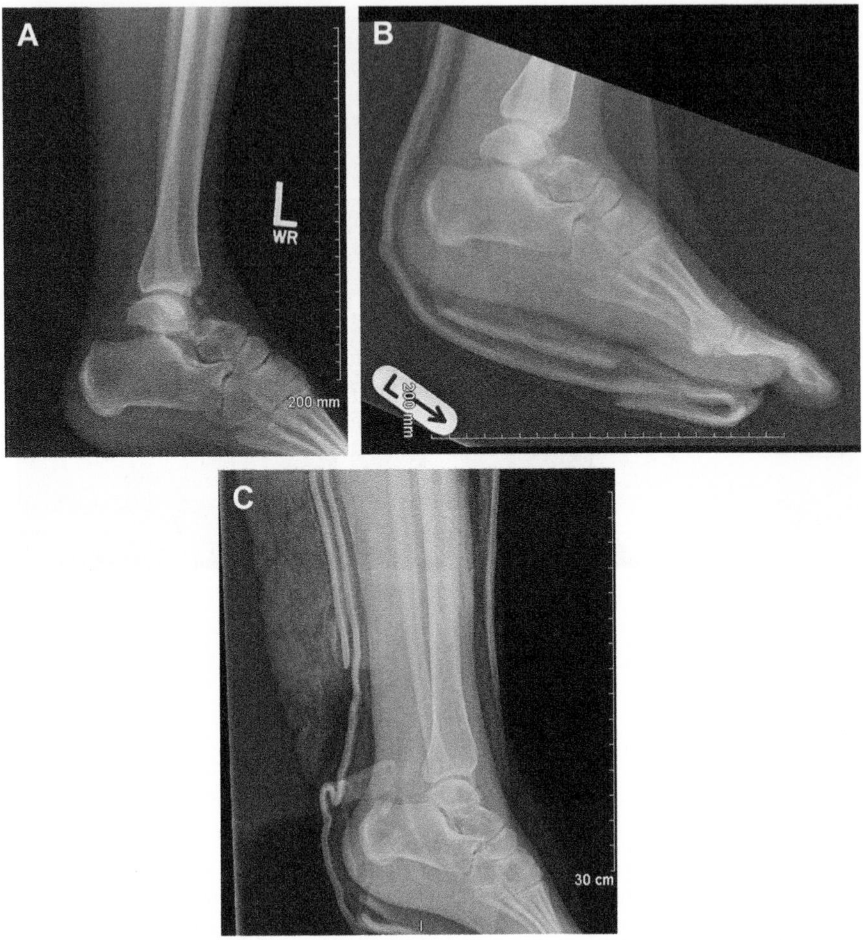

Fig. 7. (*A*) Lateral radiograph of a talar neck fracture with dislocation. (*B*) Lateral radiograph of the failed initial reduction with splint incorrectly in neutral. (*C*) Successful postreduction with splint correctly in plantarflexion. (*Courtesy of* Justin J. Fleming, DPM, American College of Foot and Ankle Surgeons, Philadelphia, PA.)

evacuation of fracture debris may help reduce post-traumatic arthrosis of the subtalar joint, a common postoperative complication. The medial incision can be, if needed, extended proximally, coursing upward in line with the coronal bisection of the medial malleolus, in instances where medial malleolar osteotomies are needed to facilitate visualization of those hybrid neck fractures that extend into the body (**Fig. 9**).

A small transversely oriented Schanz pin or intermediately sized threaded Steinman placed into the head of the talus is helpful in controlling frontal plane rotation and fracture reduction. Small wire fixation facilitates temporary stabilization of the fracture fragments before delivery of definitive fixation. These provisional wires are retrograded from medial and lateral surgical incisions oriented into the body from entry points distal to the neck fracture, adjacent to the talar head (**Fig. 10**). When possible, mini fragment plate fixation contoured adjacent to the lateral neck near the insertion of the anterior talofibular ligament facilitates delivery of stable fixation in a fanlike orientation with two screws on either side of the fracture. The real estate for fixation along the medial

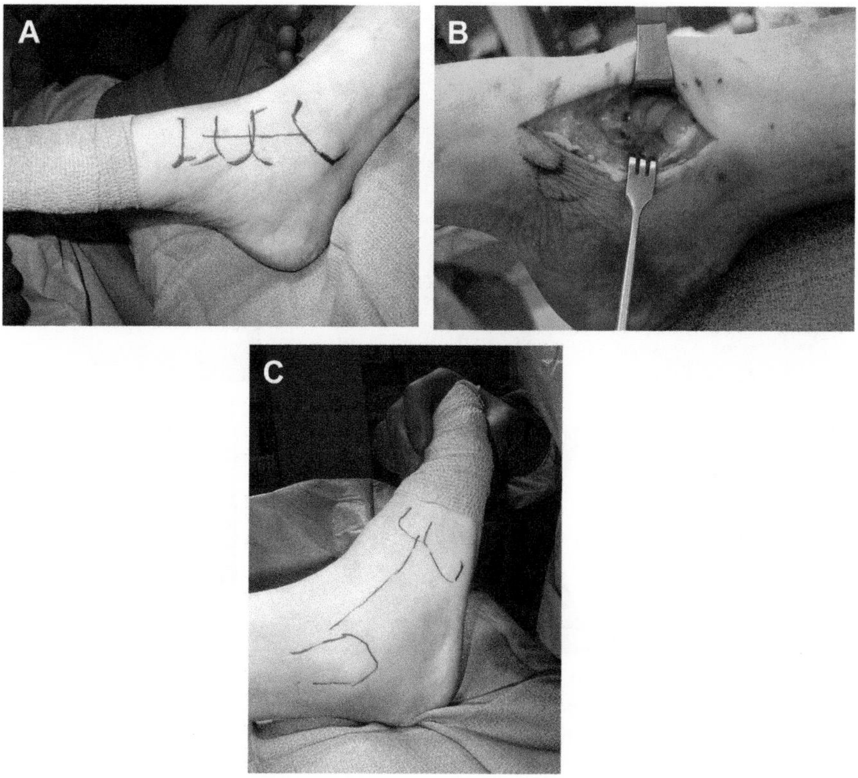

Fig. 8. Intraoperative skin marking of the planned dual incision (*A, C*) along with the intraoperative clinical picture of the medial approach (*B*). (*Courtesy of* Justin J. Fleming, DPM, American College of Foot and Ankle Surgeons, Philadelphia, PA.)

aspect of the talus is further limited. However, located just inferior to the comma-shaped facet and just distal to the deep deltoid ligament, the anatomy allows for small plate fixation if needed (**Fig. 11**). In lieu of plate fixation medially, in the absence of significant comminution, and in the presence of good cortical fracture interdigitation, mini or small fragment lag screw fixation may be delivered with the same retrograde orientation as the temporary wires, countersunk below the articular cartilage of the medial talar head (**Fig. 12**). Expected screw lengths typically span the ranges 25 mm to 40 mm. In the presence of comminution, lag screw fixation may promote varus malreduction and as such bridge plating and positional screw fixation is preferred.[25–27] Large cannulated anterograde-oriented screw placement may also be used because they have been reported to provide increased mechanical advantage. However, they require significant skill for accurate placement and avoiding catastrophic disruption of the time-consuming accurate anatomic reduction and really should be reserved for type I fractures, and minimally displaced type II fractures.[2] Furthermore, the prominent screw heads could cause posterior ankle impingement. Aggressively countersinking the screws below the chondral surface may avoid this (**Fig. 13**).

SURGICAL MANAGEMENT OF TALAR BODY FRACTURES

Traditional incisional approaches are not as uniform as with neck fractures (**Fig. 14**). Nevertheless, the aforementioned anteromedial approach with the medial malleolar

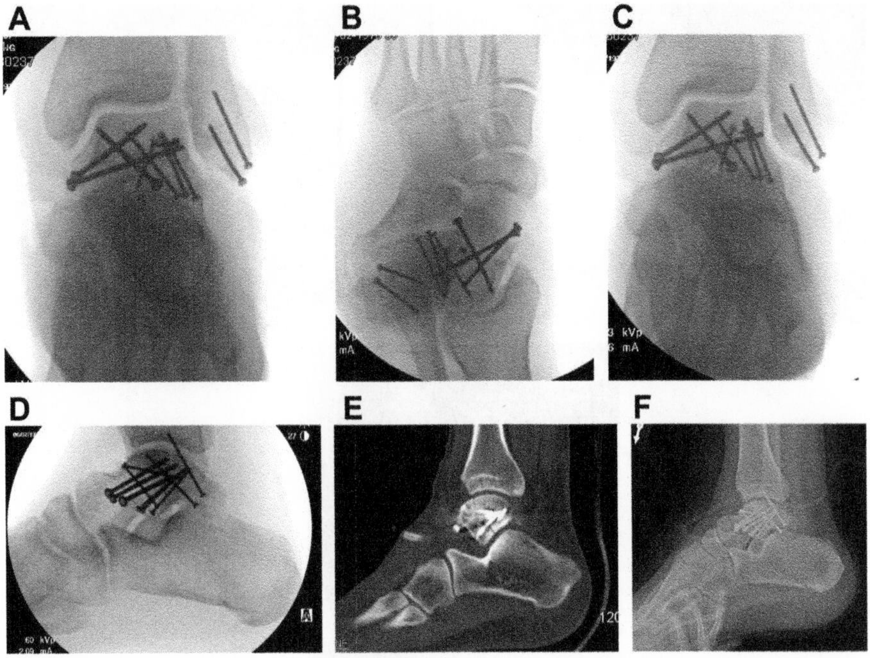

Fig. 9. (*A–F*) Preoperative and postoperative radiographs and fluoroscopic images of a hybrid talar neck/body fracture. (*Courtesy of* Justin J. Fleming, DPM, American College of Foot and Ankle Surgeons, Philadelphia, PA.)

osteotomy is useful for body fractures.[30–32] Following direct medial exposure, two screws are placed in standard Arbeitsgemeinschaft fur Osteosynthesefragen technique, before the osteotomy. The screws are placed from the inferior aspect of the medial malleolus obliquely toward the lateral tibial cortex (**Fig. 15**). The following sequence of events is important as to reduce the risk of varus malunion of the malleolus that could further complicate the recovery. An axis guidewire is placed into the medial malleolus, approximately 3.5 cm superior to the ankle plafond, perpendicular to the screw orientation toward the medial talar shoulder. The screws are then

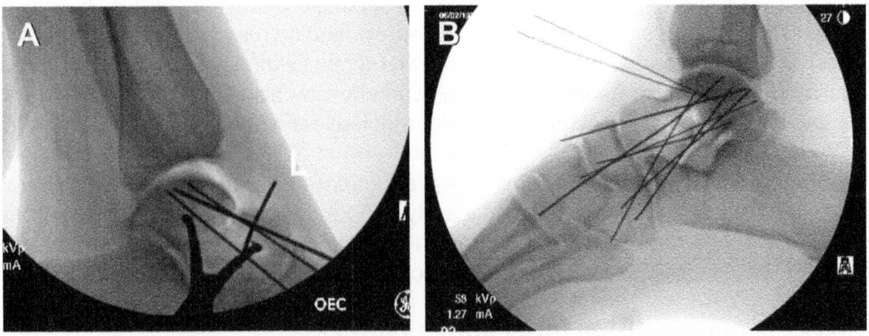

Fig. 10. (*A, B*) Intraoperative fluoroscopy films of two different talar neck fractures with two different densities of necessary wires for adequate temporary fixation. (*Courtesy of* Justin J. Fleming, DPM, American College of Foot and Ankle Surgeons, Philadelphia, PA.)

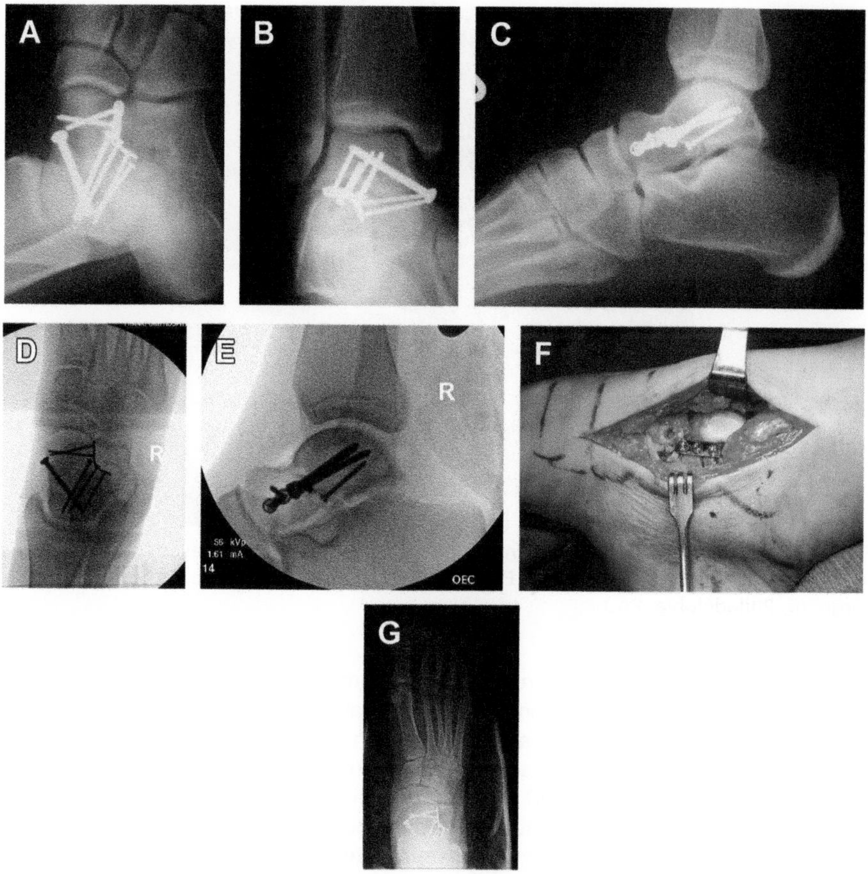

Fig. 11. (*A–G*) Intraoperative fluoroscopic and postoperative images of a talar neck fracture open reduction with plate internal fixation. (*Courtesy of* Justin J. Fleming, DPM, American College of Foot and Ankle Surgeons, Philadelphia, PA.)

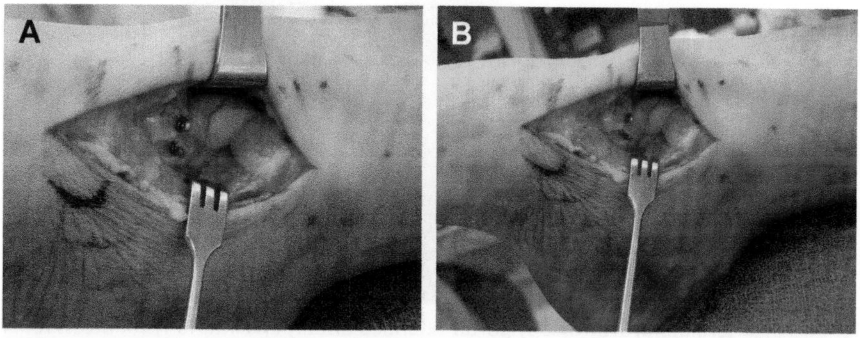

Fig. 12. (*A, B*) Medial screw fixation. (*Courtesy of* Justin J. Fleming, DPM, American College of Foot and Ankle Surgeons, Philadelphia, PA.)

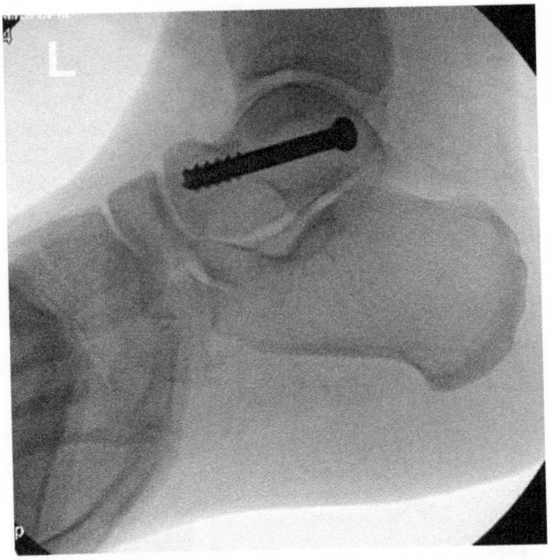

Fig. 13. The anterograde screw is countersunk well into the talus to prevent posterior ankle impingement. (*Courtesy of* Justin J. Fleming, DPM, American College of Foot and Ankle Surgeons, Philadelphia, PA.)

removed and the saw is used to create the osteotomy along the axis guide. The medial malleolus is reflected inferiorly along the deltoid ligament hinge to allow visualization of the talus trochlear. Following anatomic reduction, mini and small fragment screws countersunk below the chondral surface are recommended.

Although less common, a short transverse osteotomy of the lateral malleolus, or a short oblique osteotomy, at the level of the syndesmosis can be performed with posterior reflection when visualization of the lateral talar trochlear proves difficult.[21] In lieu of this osteotomy, sectioning the anterior talofibular ligament facilitates plantarflexion and anterior subluxation of the talus, increasing visualization. Following completion of the operations, the ligament can be repaired primarily.

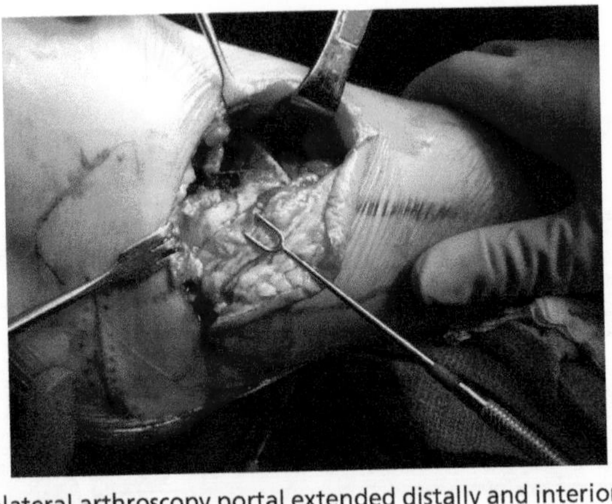

Fig. 14. An anterolateral arthroscopy portal extended distally and interiorly for access for an anterolateral talar/neck body fracture. (*Courtesy of* Justin J. Fleming, DPM, American College of Foot and Ankle Surgeons, Philadelphia, PA.)

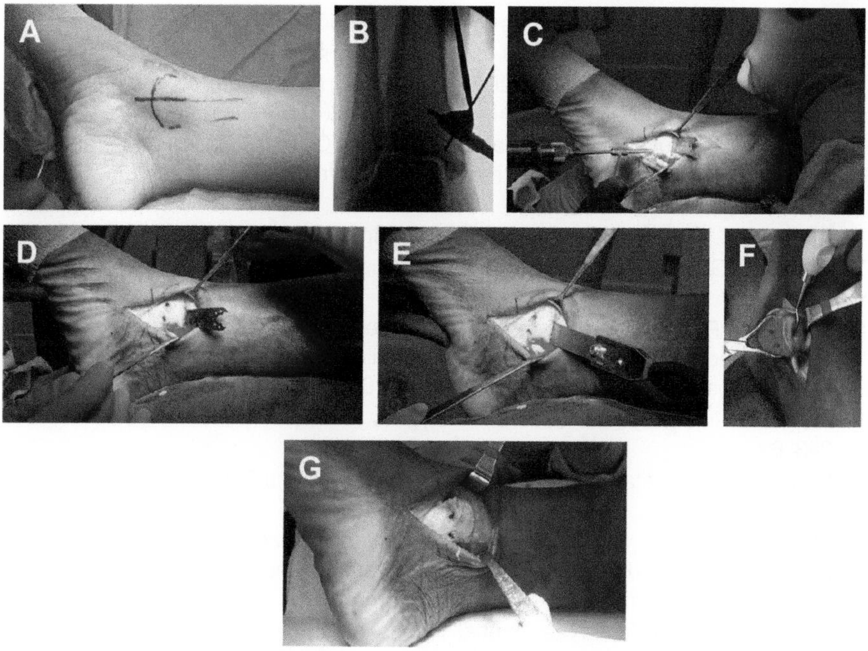

Fig. 15. (*A–G*) The medial malleolar osteotomy. (*Courtesy of* Justin J. Fleming, DPM, American College of Foot and Ankle Surgeons, Philadelphia, PA.)

As with neck fractures, temporary small wire fixation is helpful before hardware delivery. Because these fractures are wholly articular, plate fixation is never indicated even with comminuted fractures. Small mini fragment screws aggressively yet cautiously countersunk below the chondral surface is recommended. Solid screw fixation is preferred but absorbable wires may be useful in stabilizing small chondral fractures without attached subchondral bone.

SUMMARY

Fractures of the talar neck and body are difficult injuries and in the presence of significant comminution, definitive reconstruction may not always be feasible. Under these conditions, initial morphologic reconstruction with symptomatic treatment of post-traumatic arthritis at a later date should be the goal. Sanders and colleagues[31] demonstrated a near 50% need for secondary operations because of post-traumatic arthritis within 10 years of the initial injury.[33]

With little margin for error, fractures of the talar neck and body draw onto the forefront the full armamentarium of the surgeon's fracture care abilities and the respect awarded the surrounding soft tissues. A deficit in any of the previously mentioned reduces the recovery amplitude of this already difficult injury.

REFERENCES

1. Early JS. Management of fractures of the talus: body and head regions. Foot Ankle Clin 2004;9(4):709–22.
2. Abdelkafy A, Imam MA, Sokkar S, et al. Antegrade-retrograde opposing lag screws for internal fixation of simple displaced talar neck fractures. J Foot Ankle Surg 2015;54(1):23–8.

3. Dodd A, Lefaivre KA. Outcomes of talar neck fractures: a systematic review and meta-analysis. J Orthop Trauma 2015;29(5):210–5.
4. Halvorson JJ, Winter SB, Teasdall RD, et al. Talar neck fractures: a systematic review of the literature. J Foot Ankle Surg 2013;52(1):56–61.
5. Lindvall E, Haidukewych G, Dipasquale T, et al. Open reduction and stable fixation of isolated, displaced talar neck and body fractures. J Bone Joint Surg Am 2004;86(10):2229–34.
6. Rammelt S, Zwipp H. Talar neck and body fractures. Injury 2009;40(2):120–35.
7. Hawkins LG. Fractures of the neck of the talus. J Bone Joint Surg Am 1970;52(5): 991–1002.
8. Vallier HA, Reichard SG, Boyd AJ, et al. A new look at the Hawkins classification for talar neck fractures: which features of injury and treatment are predictive of osteonecrosis? J Bone Joint Surg Am 2014;96(3):192–7.
9. Kleiger B. Injuries of the talus and its joints. Clin Orthop Relat Res 1976;(121): 243–62.
10. Mulfinger GL, Trueta J. The blood supply of the talus. J Bone Joint Surg Br 1970; 52(1):160–7.
11. Miller AN, Prasarn ML, Dyke JP, et al. Quantitative assessment of the vascularity of the talus with gadolinium-enhanced magnetic resonance imaging. J Bone Joint Surg Am 2011;93(12):1116–21.
12. Prasarn ML, Miller AN, Dyke JP, et al. Arterial anatomy of the talus: a cadaver and gadolinium-enhanced MRI study. Foot Ankle Int 2010;31(11):987–93.
13. Metzger MJ, Levin JS, Clancy JT. Talar neck fractures and rates of avascular necrosis. J Foot Ankle Surg 1999;38(2):154–62.
14. Adelaar RS, Madrian JR. Avascular necrosis of the talus. Orthop Clin North Am 2004;35(3):383–95.
15. Vallier HA, Nork SE, Barei DP, et al. Talar neck fractures: results and outcomes. J Bone Joint Surg Am 2004;86(8):1616–24.
16. Thordarson DB, Triffon MJ, Terk MR. Magnetic resonance imaging to detect avascular necrosis after open reduction and internal fixation of talar neck fractures. Foot Ankle Int 1996;17(12):742–7.
17. Sneppen O, Christensen SB, Krogsøe O, et al. Fractures of the body of the talus. Acta Orthop Scand 1977;48(3):317–24.
18. Peterson L, Romanus B, Dahlberg E. Fracture of the collum tali: an experimental study. J Biomech 1976;9(4):277–9.
19. Sarrafian SK. Anatomy of the foot and ankle. 2nd edition. Philadelphia: Lippincott; 1993.
20. Sanders R, Lindvall E. Fractures and fracture-dislocations of the talus. In: Coughlin MJ, Mann RA, Saltzman CL, editors. Surgery of the foot and ankle. 8th edition. Philadelphia: Mosby; 2007. p. 2075–136.
21. Rush SM, Hamilton GA. Talus fractures: surgical principles. Clin Podiatr Med Surg 2009;26(1):91–103.
22. Furlong J, Morrison WB, Carrino JA. Imaging of the talus. Foot Ankle Clin 2004; 9(4):685–701.
23. Early JS. Talus fracture management. Foot Ankle Clin 2008;13(4):635–57.
24. Marceroli MA, Wong C, Sanders RW, et al. Treatment of comminuted talar neck fractures with use of minifragment plating. J Orthop Trauma 2016;30(10):572–8.
25. Barg A, Suter T, Nickisch F, et al. Osteotomies of the talar neck for posttraumatic malalignment. Foot Ankle Clin 2016;21(1):77–93.

26. Daniels TR, Smith JW, Ross TI. Varus malalignment of the talar neck. Its effect on the position of the foot and on subtalar motion. J Bone Joint Surg Am 1996; 78(10):1559–67.
27. Sangeorzan BJ, Wagner UA, Harrington RM, et al. Contact characteristics of the subtalar joint: the effect of talar neck misalignment. J Orthop Res 1992;10(4): 544–51.
28. Summers NJ, Murdoch MM. Fractures of the talus: a comprehensive review. Clin Podiatr Med Surg 2012;29(2):187–203.
29. Léduc S, Clare MP, Laflamme GY, et al. Posttraumatic avascular necrosis of the talus. Foot Ankle Clin 2008;13(4):753–65.
30. Schuberth JM, Rush SM, Jennings MM. Talar fractures. In: Southerland JT, Boberg JS, Downey MS, et al, editors. Mcglamry's comprehensive textbook of foot and ankle surgery. 4th edition. Philadelphia: Lippincott Williams & Wilkins; 2013. p. 1707–38.
31. Sanders DW, Busam M, Hattwick E, et al. Functional outcomes after talar neck fractures. J Orthop Trauma 2004;18(5):265–70.
32. Mann RA. Arthrodesis of the foot and ankle. In: Coughlin MJ, Mann RA, Saltzman CL, editors. Surgery of the foot and ankle. 8th edition. Philadelphia: Mosby; 2007. p. 1087–123.
33. Fournier A, Barba N, Steiger V, et al. Total talar fracture – long-term results of internal fixation of talar fractures. A multicentric study of 114 cases. Orthop Traumatol Surg Res 2012;98(4 Suppl):s48–55.

Paradigm Shift for the Surgical Management of Calcaneal Fractures?

Spencer J. Monaco, DPM[a], Michael Calderone, DPM[a], Justin J. Fleming, DPM[b,*]

KEYWORDS

- Calcaneal fracture • Sinus tarsi approach • Primary arthrodesis

KEY POINTS

- Sinus tarsi approach offers a less invasive approach to operative reduction of calcaneal fractures with lower complications rates.
- Calcaneal fractures are more common in men, who are typically in the industrial profession.
- The literature continues to support surgical intervention for displaced intraarticular calcaneal fractures; however, these injuries can still be managed nonoperatively in certain clinical scenarios.
- The article focuses on the surgical management of intraarticular calcaneal fractures and highlights the sinus tarsi approach.

THE BASICS

Understanding the osseous anatomy is paramount when treating these fractures surgically.[1–3] Routine plain radiographs are standard and measured angles, such as the Böhler angle and the crucial angle of Gissane, are used to assess the degree of injury. Plain radiographs include anteroposterior, medial oblique, lateral, and calcaneal axial views of the foot. Based on plain radiographs, Essex-Lopresti[3] divides calcaneal fractures into tongue-type and joint-depression. Typically, the crucial angle of Gissane is between 125° to 140° and is increased with intraarticular fractures (>145°). The Böhler angle is normally between 25° and 40°, and will decrease with intraarticular pathologic abnormality (**Fig. 1**). A computed tomography (CT) scan is mandatory to further evaluate the degree of intraarticular injury. High-resolution 3-dimensional reconstructed images are useful for preoperative planning and further understanding

Disclosure: Dr J.J. Fleming is a consultant for Arthrex Inc and Stryker Orthopedics. Other authors have nothing to disclose.
[a] Premier Orthopaedics, 400 McFarlan Road, Suite 100, Kennett Square, PA 19348, USA; [b] University Orthopaedic Associates, 2 World's Fair Drive, Somerset, NJ 08873, USA
* Corresponding author.
E-mail address: flemingjmak@gmail.com

Clin Podiatr Med Surg 35 (2018) 175–182
https://doi.org/10.1016/j.cpm.2017.12.002
podiatric.theclinics.com

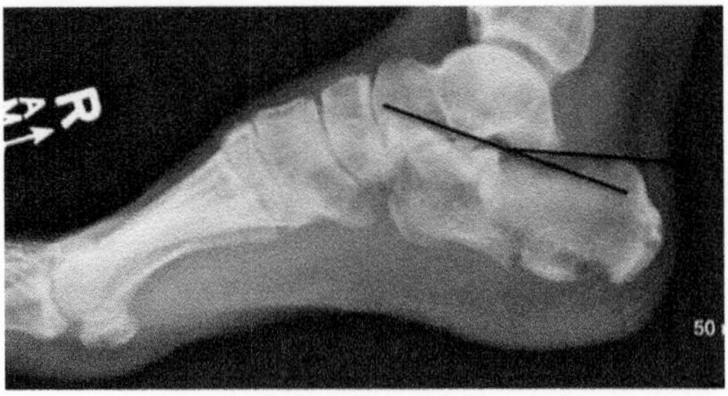

Fig. 1. Calcaneal joint depression fracture illustrating a decrease in Böhler angle.

of fracture patterns. The Sanders classification system is also routinely used to classify the injury ranging for nondisplaced injuries (type-I) to severely comminuted fractures (type-IV).[4] Generally, as the severity of the injury increases, the fractures become more complex and it becomes difficult to restore the normal osseous anatomy and articular joints. Surgical approaches vary for calcaneal open reduction internal fixation (ORIF) and can range from minimally invasive techniques, such as percutaneous incisions, to large lateral extensile approaches. In select cases of Sanders type-III and type-IV fractures, ORIF combined with primary subtalar joint arthrodesis may be indicated.

SURGICAL GOALS

With proper evaluation of plain radiographs and CT scans, typical fracture patterns are observed. Articular fractures, posterior facet depression, lateral wall displacement, calcaneal length shortening, varus orientation, and lateralization of the calcaneal body are commonly identified (**Box 1**). The surgeon must review all images thoroughly and the injury must be approached in a stepwise fashion to restore the osseous anatomy. Various approaches have been described in the literature to address these issues, including the lateral extensile incision, the sinus tarsi incision, and percutaneous approaches.

TRADITIONAL LATERAL EXTENSILE APPROACH

Traditional approaches include large incisions on the lateral aspect of the ankle and hindfoot, which gives the surgeon an excellent view of the fractures.[5] This approach will provide visualization of the subtalar and calcaneocuboid joints, which facilitates joint restoration. The extended lateral approach aids in the understanding of this complex injury and can help the surgeon conceptualize the fracture pattern. Once the fractures are reduced, the varus and translation restored, and the joint is reconstructed, fixation can be potentially easier through this type of incision. The lateral wall of the

Box 1
Surgical goals of calcaneal open reduction internal fixation

Surgical goals

- Restore calcaneal length
- Remove varus deformity
- Translate posterior tuberosity medially
- Restore calcaneal width
- Address depression of posterior facet
- Restore the joint or joints

calcaneus is relatively flat and is most suitable for plating options.[6] With improved visualization through a larger extended incision come the potential risks associated with it. The risks with this approach have historically been related to the wound and the nerve. The rate of wound complications following the extended lateral approach has been reported as up to 30% of patients.[7] Before performing this type of incision, Bibbo and colleagues[8] revealed the importance in identifying proper vascularity of the large lateral flap by using a hand-held Doppler. The lateral calcaneal artery must be patent before using this incision to decrease the dreaded complications of wound healing. Although this incision is extremely utilitarian and safe, to address this injury other approaches are becoming more desirable due to the morbidity of a traditional lateral extensile incision. Restoring the range of motion of the subtalar joint postoperatively may also be more challenging when an extended lateral approach is used because of soft tissue adhesions and scarring, although this has not been fully investigated in the literature owing to its inherit challenges.

PERCUTANEOUS APPROACH

Percutaneous approaches in addressing certain fracture patterns of calcaneal fractures remain viable options. The benefits of this approach include decreases in operative time, wound complications, nerve injury, and postoperative stiffness. The challenges with this approach include limited exposure of the fracture, the potential inability to fully restore the normal osseous anatomy and more difficulty in placing rigid internal fixation. Arthroscopic assistance may help aid the surgeon in restoring the articular surface. This approach better serves less complex calcaneal fractures, typically Sanders type II and tongue-type fractures. Rammelt and colleagues[9] reviewed 61 patients who underwent a percutaneous approach for Sanders type II calcaneal fractures. In 33 of the 61 fractures treated, anatomic reduction was confirmed with arthroscopy and served as the basis of the review. Of the 33 patients treated with a percutaneous approach, 24 patients (73%) were followed for a minimum of 24 months. The patient cohort consisted of Sanders type IIA and type IIB fractures. Arthroscopic assistance was not performed in Sanders type IIC fractures and was not included in the 33 patients reviewed. The American Orthopedic Foot and Ankle Society ankle-hindfoot score at final follow-up was 91.2. The investigators concluded that a percutaneous approach for moderately displaced type II fractures provided adequate control over anatomic joint reduction with either subtalar joint arthroscopy or high-resolution (3-dimensional) fluoroscopy.

Percutaneous approaches clearly have a role with surgically managing calcaneal joint depression fractures; however, this approach must be carefully selected for mild to moderately displaced fractures.

SINUS TARSI APPROACH

The sinus tarsi incision has been gaining popularity due to the potential decrease in postoperative complications, including hematoma formation, wound complications, infection, need for further surgery, and sural nerve injury.[10–12] Kline and colleagues[13] retrospectively reviewed 112 intraarticular calcaneal fractures. Seventy-nine fractures were treated with a lateral extensile approach versus 33 fractures with a minimally invasive approach based on surgeon's preface. Charts and radiographs were reviewed specifically for wound complications and the need for further surgery. Overall, the lateral extensile approach was found to have a wound complication rate of 29% versus 6% in the minimally invasive group. A further analysis was performed on 47 patients to include a research follow-up visit for radiographs, clinical examination, and quality-of-life questionnaires (Short Form-36 [SF-36], Foot Function Index [FFI], and visual analog scale [VAS] pain). Overall, 84% of the patients in the extensile group were satisfied versus 94% in the minimally invasive group. Yeo and colleagues[14] performed a retrospective review on 100 patients with a displaced intraarticular calcaneal fracture. There was an equal distribution in Sanders type-II and type-III fracture patterns. Of the 100 patients, 60 were treated with a lateral extensile approach compared with 40 patients with a sinus tarsi approach. All patients were evaluated for both clinical and radiographic review. There were no statistical differences found when comparing the groups; however, wound complication rates were 13.3% in the extensile group and 5% in the sinus tarsi group. In 2011, a systematic review was performed to identify studies evaluating a sinus tarsi or modified sinus tarsi approach for the treatment of displaced intraarticular calcaneal fractures. Eight case series reporting on 256 patients were included. Overall, 75% of the patients managed with this approach had good to excellent outcomes. Minor wound complications were observed in 4.1%. The investigator concluded that the sinus tarsi approach compares similarly or favorably to the extended lateral extensile approach.[15]

This approach is typically started 1 cm inferior to the lateral malleolus and is extended toward the calcaneocuboid joint. This allows visualization of both the subtalar and calcaneocuboid joints. Again, a stepwise approach is used to restore the calcaneal

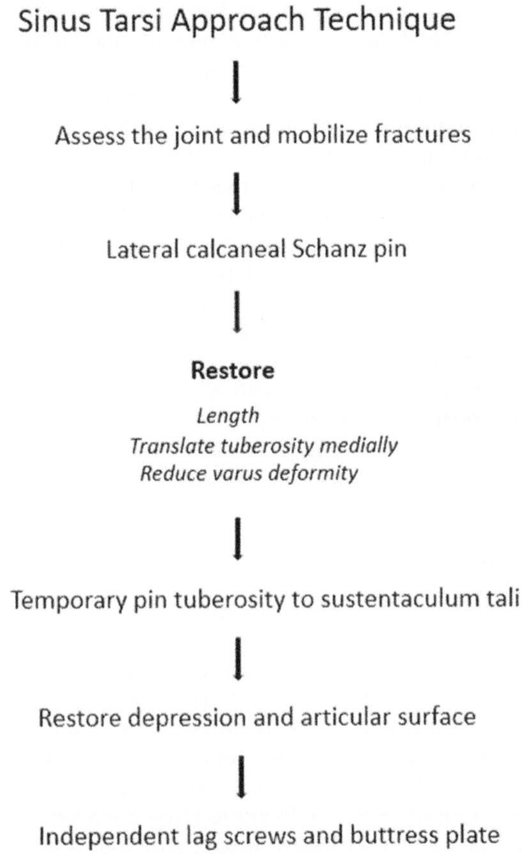
Sinus Tarsi Approach Technique
Assess the joint and mobilize fractures
Lateral calcaneal Schanz pin
Restore
Length
Translate tuberosity medially
Reduce varus deformity
Temporary pin tuberosity to sustentaculum tali
Restore depression and articular surface
Independent lag screws and buttress plate

Fig. 2. Stepwise approach for calcaneal ORIF.

length, translate the posterior tuberosity medially, remove the varus deformity, and restore the articular surface of the posterior facet and calcaneocuboid joint (**Fig. 2**). Screws can independently be placed to lag across the posterior facet into the sustentaculum tali; rim plate techniques may be performed, if necessary; and a lateral buttress plate can be placed.

PREFERRED SINUS TARSI TECHNIQUE

Case 1

A 52-year-old man fell from a height of approximately 8 feet. Plain radiographs revealed an intraarticular calcaneal joint depression fracture. CT scans demonstrated a Sanders type II A fracture. The patient was placed in the lateral decubitus position on a bean bag. A modified sinus tarsi approach was used (**Fig. 3**). A percutaneous 5-mm Schanz pin was placed from lateral to medial to manually restore calcaneal length, varus deformity, and translation. This was followed by temporary pinning into the

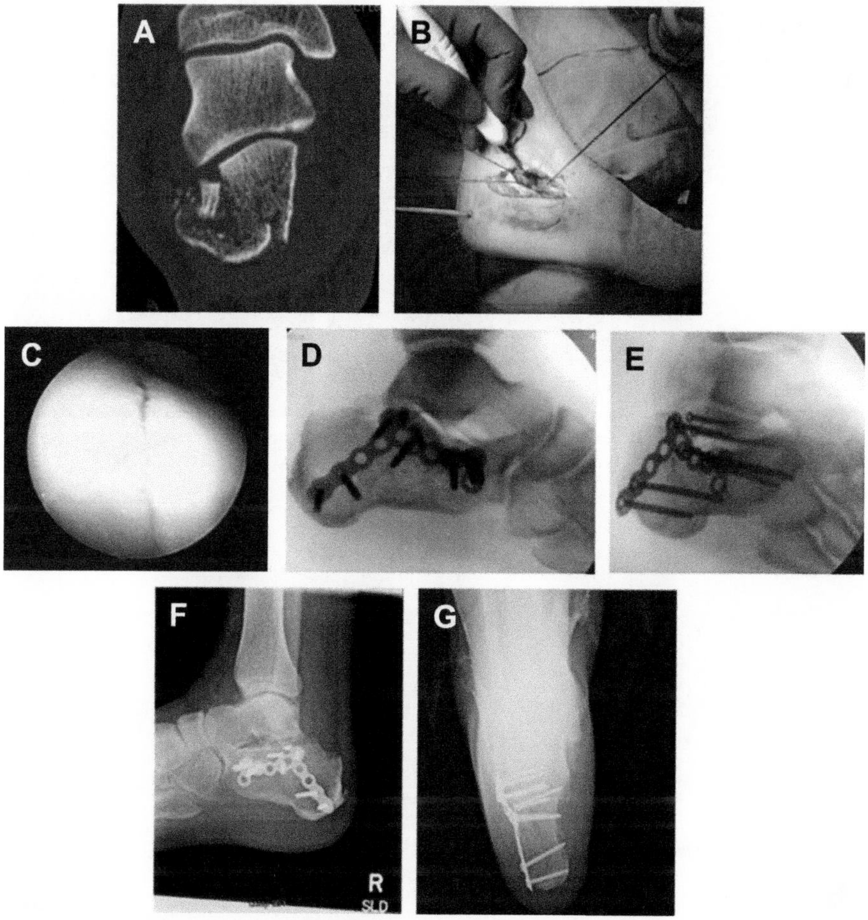

Fig. 3. Lateral posterior facet joint depression (*A*). Sinus tarsi approach (*B*). Arthroscopic evaluation of articular fracture reduction (*C*). Lateral and modified Broden intraoperative fluoroscopic images confirming reduction (*D* and *E*). Postoperative lateral and calcaneal axial images (*F* and *G*).

sustentaculum tali. A calcaneal axial image was obtained to ensure reduction of the tuberosity. The joint was then reconstructed. Two independent 3.0-mm lag screws were placed from lateral to medial into the sustentaculum tali. Arthroscopic assessment added in reduction of the posterior facet, specifically assessing the posterior aspect, which is often difficult to visualize through a sinus tarsi incision. An anatomic lateral calcaneal plate was used to buttress and maintain the posterior tuberosity, posterior facet, and anterior calcaneus. A subperiosteal tunnel is made through the sinus tarsi incision to place the plate posteriorly percutaneous, ensuring that the plate was placed lateral to the lateral calcaneal wall. Cancellous allograft was used to backfill any osseous void.

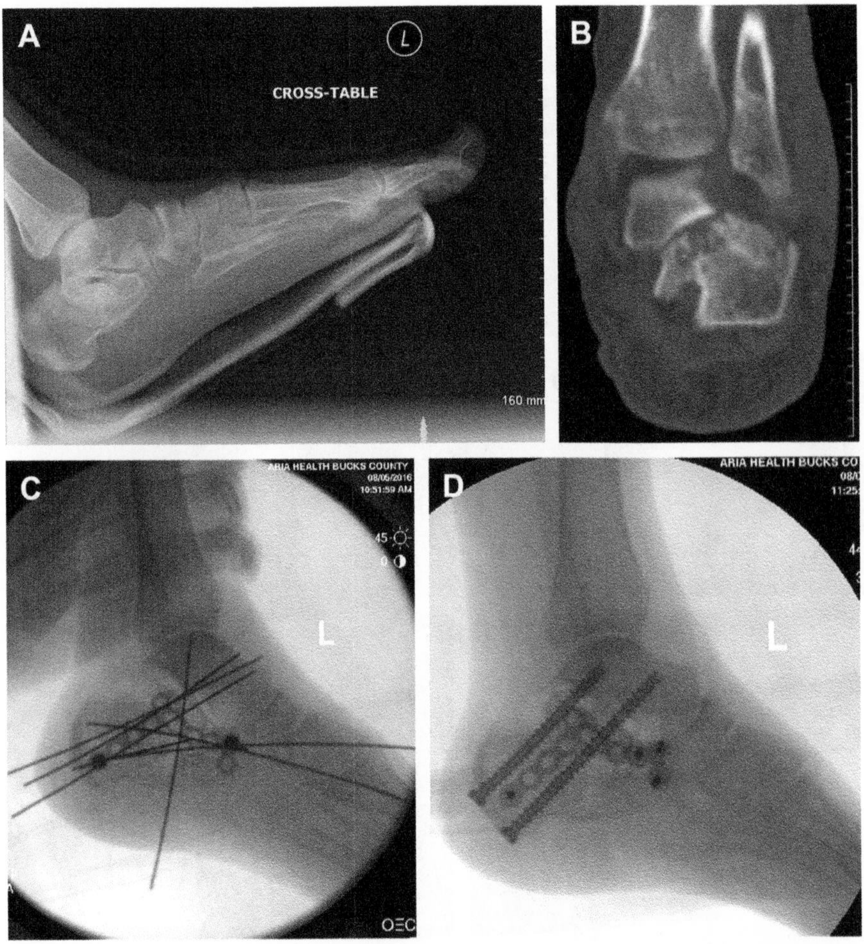

Fig. 4. (*A*) Closed joint depression calcaneal fracture. (*B*) Coronal CT image demonstrating comminution and osteochondral deformation. (*C*) Intraoperative lateral radiograph showing restoration or calcaneal height and length. (*D*) Lateral radiograph showing ORIF plus primary arthrodesis of the subtalar joint.

Case 2

A 36-year-old woman sustained 2 bilateral closed calcaneal fractures in a motor vehicle accident. The patient underwent operative repair for both injuries when the soft tissue envelope was supportive. Due to the preoperative imaging findings and intraoperative chondral damage, primary arthrodesis was performed in addition to ORIF. Femoral head bone graft allograft was used to restore the hindfoot height. Fully threaded screws and a low-profile lateral plate were placed to maintain surgical reduction (**Fig. 4**).

SUMMARY

Calcaneal fractures are inherently difficult fractures and are associated with a high degree of associated morbidity. Surgical management for these injuries is now considered the gold standard in most clinical scenarios. The lateral extensile approach remains a widely used and accepted approach for addressing these challenging fractures. As surgeon understanding and techniques evolve, arthroscopic assistance and percutaneous and sinus tarsi approaches will continue to advance surgical management. The sinus tarsi approach provides good visualization of the posterior facet and facilitates anatomic reduction and a corridor for appropriate internal fixation with a potential decrease in wound and nerve complications.

REFERENCES

1. Potter MQ, Nunley JA. Long-term functional outcomes after operative treatment for intra-articular fractures of the calcaneus. J Bone Joint Surg Am 2009;91:1854–60.
2. Razik A, Harris M, Trompeter A. Calcaneal fracture: where are we now? Strategies Trauma Limb Reconstr 2017. [Epub ahead of print].
3. Essex-Lopresti P. The mechanism, reduction technique, and results in fractures of the os calcis. Br J Surg 1952;39(157):395–419.
4. Sanders R, Fortin P, DiPasquale T, et al. Operative treatment in 120 displaced intraarticular calcaneal fractures. Results using a prognostic computed tomography scan classification. Clin Orthop Relat Res 1993;290:87–95.
5. Buckley R, Tough S, McCormack R, et al. Operative compared with nonoperative treatment of displaced intra-articular calcaneal fractures. J Bone Joint Surg Am 2002;84:1733–44.
6. Benirschke SK, Sangeorzan BL. Extensive intra-articular fractures of the foot: surgical management of calcaneal fractures. Clin Orthop Relat Res 1993;29:128–34.
7. Abidi NA, Dhawan S, Gruen GS, et al. Wound-healing risk factors after open reduction and internal fixation of calcaneal fractures. Foot Ankle Int 1998;19:856–86.
8. Bibbo C, Ehrlich DA, Nguyen HM, et al. Low wound complications rates for the lateral extensile approach for calcaneal ORIF when the lateral calcaneal artery is patent. Foot Ankle Int 2014;35:650–6.
9. Rammelt S, Heineck J, Barthel S, et al. Percutaneous fixation of intraarticular calcaneus fractures. Tech Foot Ankle Surg 2009;8:70–6.
10. Al-Mudhaffar M. Wound complications following operative fixation of calcaneal fracture. Injury 2009;31:461–4.
11. Harvey EJ, Grujic L, Early JS, et al. Morbidity associated with ORIF of intra-articular calcaneus fractures using a lateral approach. Foot Ankle Int 2001;11:868–73.

12. Benirschke SK, Kramer PA. Wound healing complications in closed and open calcaneal fractures. J Orthop Trauma 2004;18:1–6.
13. Kline AJ, Anderson RB, Davis WH, et al. Minimally invasive technique versus an extensile lateral approach for intra-articular calcaneal fractures. Foot Ankle Int 2013;34:773–80.
14. Yeo H, Cho H, Lee K. Comparison of two surgical approaches for displaced intra-articular calcaneal fractures: sinus tarsi versus extensile lateral approach. BMC Musculoskelet Disord 2015;16:63.
15. Schepers T. The sinus tarsi approach in displaced intra-articular calcaneal fractures: a systemic review. Int Orthop 2011;35:697–703.

Role for Primary Repair of Deltoid Ligament Complex in Ankle Fractures

Ryan B. Rigby, DPM[a,*], Ryan T. Scott, DPM[b]

KEYWORDS

• Ankle • Deltoid • Fracture • Primary • Acute

KEY POINTS

- Deltoid injuries of varying degrees often occur in association with ankle fractures; partial or complete deltoid tears may lead to persistent instability.
- Medial ankle ligament instability is not tolerated well and may lead to long-term negative changes in the ankle joint.
- Stress views are often necessary to determine the extent of deltoid injury. Gravity stress views are as effective as manual stress.
- Acute deltoid injuries may be evaluated and repaired using arthroscopy or an open approach.
- Surgeons should consider primary repair of acute deltoid injuries that demonstrate instability following fracture stabilization.

INTRODUCTION

Ankle fractures may be mistaken for purely bony injuries. Surgeons, however, understand the imperative role periarticular ligamentous structures play in the functionality of the ankle joint. Much work has been done to better understand the ankle mortise and establish ideal methods for stabilizing the distal syndesmosis. Traditionally, surgeons have a low threshold for placing fixation at the syndesmosis itself, while leaving the known deltoid injury to heal without repair. With the growing interest in joint-sparing procedures, such as total ankle replacement, surgeons are encountering more and more ligamentous insufficiency complicating such procedures. For this and other reasons, a growing trend toward performing primary repair of the concomitant ligamentous injuries associated with ankle fractures is occurring.

Disclosure: The authors have nothing to disclose.
[a] Logan Regional Orthopedics, 1350 North 500 East, Logan, UT 84321, USA; [b] CORE Institute, 9305 West Thomas Road #305, Phoenix, AZ 85023, USA
* Corresponding author.
E-mail address: ryan.rigby@imail.org

Clin Podiatr Med Surg 35 (2018) 183–197
https://doi.org/10.1016/j.cpm.2017.12.003
podiatric.theclinics.com

ANATOMY AND PURPOSE

The deltoid ligament complex is a multilayer, multiband structure linking and providing support to the ankle, subtalar, and talonavicular joints by spanning the medial malleolus, talus, calcaneus, and navicular bones. Ultimately, the deltoid provides peritalar stability, holding the ankle within the mortise by limiting both rotational and translational forces. The role of the superficial component is to resist eversional forces of the ankle and subtalar joint. The deep ligaments restrain external rotation, as well as lateral translation of the talus.[1] The superficial component lies deep to the posterior tibial tendon whose deep sheath often is incorporated with the superficial deltoid. A thin layer of adipose tissue may interpose between the superficial and deep ligaments. Campbell and colleagues[1] performed a cadaveric analysis of the individual bands of the deltoid complex. Although they found small variations, there were certain consistencies found in each specimen. The deep layer typically consists of the posterior tibiotalar and anterior tibiotalar with the posterior being the larger more robust. The tibionavicular, tibiospring, tibiocalcaneal, and superficial posterior tibiotalar make up the superficial complex.[2]

BACKGROUND OR HISTORY

Controversy in Deltoid Repair

Few studies from the nineteenth century evaluating ankle fracture treatment promoted that repair of the deltoid was necessary. Most studies from this time suggest there is no need to repair the deltoid.[3–10] These studies set the trend for surgeons to be comfortable in leaving the deltoid injury to heal without repair. Unfortunately, by current standards, such studies are low-powered and greatly flawed. For example, Baird and Jackson,[3] in their 1987 paper, "Fractures of the Distal Part of the Fibula with Associated Disruption of the Deltoid Ligament. Treatment Without Repair of the Deltoid," promoted that exploration of the medial side of the ankle and repair of the deltoid ligament was not necessary unless reduction of the lateral malleolus fails to reduce the talus within the ankle mortise. It should be recognized that, although this was a good study for its time, it is now recognized as a relatively low-powered study because of small sample size, significant loss of patient follow-up, being single-blinded, and having no standardized scoring system. When considering whether deltoid repair is necessary, it is imperative surgeons make such decisions based on current literature and not previous historical trends.

Why Repair?

Standard treatment of ankle fractures includes reapproximation of fibula length, restoration of the ankle mortise, and rigid fixation. Long-term stability depends on appropriate balancing of the osseous and ligamentous structures. In order for this to occur, both the osseous structures, as well as the ligamentous ankle stabilizers, must heal not only with integrity but also adequate tension. The deltoid is arguably one of the most important stabilizers of the ankle mortise.[11,12] In bimalleolar equivalent or greater injuries the deltoid may be partially or completely torn. Partial injuries typically involve the anterior aspect of the deltoid complex and, depending on the severity, may be found to unveil instability of the mortise in varying degrees.[12–16] A medial malleolus fracture does not rule out deltoid injury because medial injuries may involve both ligamentous and osseous components.[9,16–18] Typically, supramalleolar medial malleolus fractures will spare the deltoid. It is important to be aware that fixation of smaller anterior medial malleolus fractures, or intercollicular fractures, containing the superficial deltoid could also involve deep deltoid disruption. Therefore, it is important to stress evaluate the medial ankle after fixation of such fractures to assess for residual instability.

Complete disruptions are obviously are more likely to be unstable and include both superficial and the deep deltoid complex (**Fig. 1**). If medial instability is identified preoperatively or intraoperatively, there is inherent risk of this persisting through the recovery period and, unfortunately, resulting in chronic instability if left untreated. When this occurs, patients often complain of a sensation of giving way on the inside of the ankle with stairs or uneven ground.[13,14] Over time, the relationship between the talus and tibia may be compromised with the development of incongruent valgus tilting. Such malalignment of the joint may lead to posttraumatic ankle arthrosis, causing pain and decreased mobility, which potentially may require further surgical procedures[15] (**Fig. 2**).

Although frequently debated, many investigators advocate for primary repair of the deltoid after intraoperative assessment if instability persists or if the deltoid rupture blocks reduction because of interposition.[12,13,19–22] Many investigators who advocate for deltoid repair seem to do so because a portion of patients in whom the fibula is repaired without deltoid treatment subsequently seem to persistent with medial ankle pain or instability, or develop malalignment leading to arthrosis of the joint.[12,23–26]

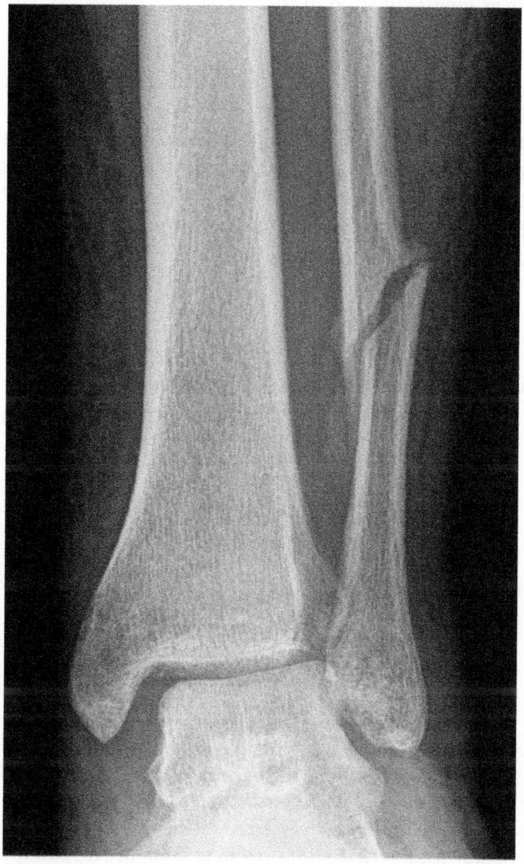

Fig. 1. Obvious complete disruption of the medial deltoid complex in association with a severe ankle dislocation and fibula fracture.

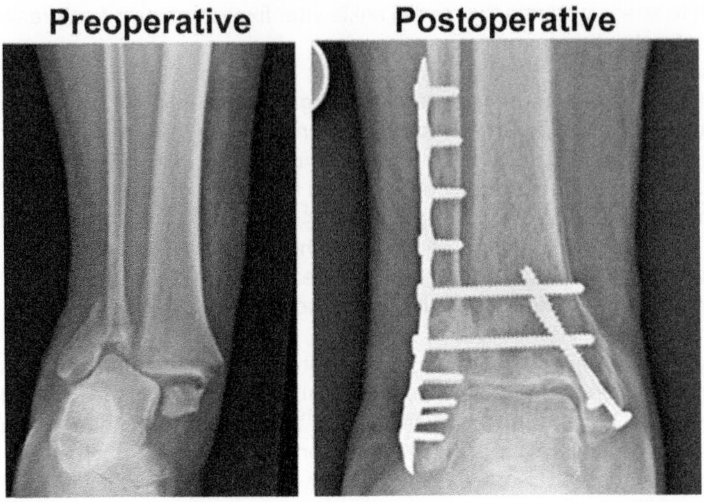

Fig. 2. Preoperative radiograph and postoperative radiograph demonstrates valgus deformity development likely secondary to insufficient deltoid. The deltoid was not primarily repaired or stressed after medial fixation in this patient.

Small amounts of instability are not well tolerated in the medial ankle. Femino and colleagues[26] described how medial deltoid insufficiency may create subtle rotatory subluxation of the talus during the late swing phase. During this time, the hindfoot is in a varus position and, as heel strike occurs, a valgus thrust is placed on the hindfoot, reducing the talus internally back into position.[27] The cumulative effect of this additional rotatory strain over time on the tibiotalar chondrocytes certainly could be a factor leading to posttraumatic arthrosis (**Fig. 3**).

IMAGING

Radiographs

A radiograph of the ankle may or may not suggest injury to the deltoid. The standard 3 views of the ankle are mandatory for ankle fracture. Typically, these are obtained while

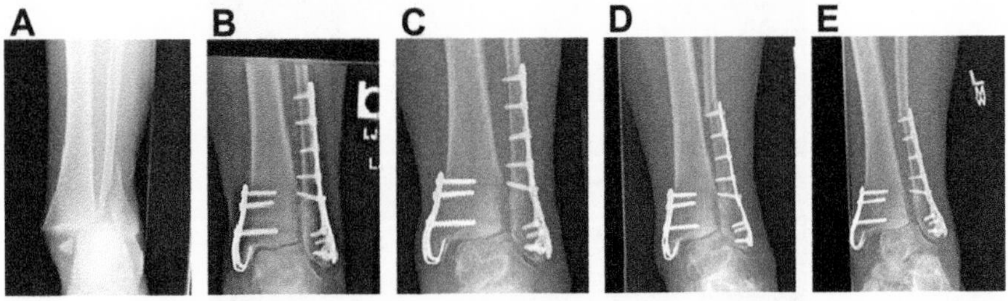

Fig. 3. (*A*) Preoperative radiograph shows bimalleolar ankle fracture. (*B*) Initial postoperative radiograph demonstrates no signs of medial clear space or deltoid insufficiency. According to the operative report, the syndesmosis was stressed and found to be stable. The deltoid, according to the report, was not repaired nor stressed intraoperatively. (*C*) Six weeks postoperative radiograph unveils medial instability. (*D*) Nine weeks postoperative radiograph with new fibula fracture developing at the proximal aspect of the plate. (*E*) At twelve weeks there appears to be syndesmosis widening in association with the new fibula fracture, and medial ankle instability.

the patient is nonweightbearing because of the fractures. For proximal fibula fractures, such as Maisonneuve-type injuries, weightbearing films are helpful if the patient can tolerate the weight.[28] Most attention is given to the medial clear space when inspecting for deltoid injury. In more subtle injuries, the medial clear space is compared with the perpendicular tibiotalar joint line and should normally be within 1 mm of this measurement.

Stress Radiographs

Both manual and gravity stress views have been used to assess the integrity of the deltoid.[29] Initial radiographs, whether weightbearing or nonweightbearing, may appear negative for signs of deltoid compromise. If the patient has medial tenderness, swelling, and bruising, further imaging beyond a standard radiograph is indicated, starting with stress radiograph. If a medial malleolus fracture is present stress, radiographs are typically unnecessary preoperatively; however, the deltoid should be stressed postfixation placement intraoperatively. Leba and colleagues[29] compared manual versus gravity stress images and found gravity stress views were comparable to manual stress for isolated fibula fractures. Gravity stress images, however, were superior because of the lack of radiation exposure to the physician, along with the ability to perform the examination without the physician being present.[30–34] It is more important to achieve adequate external rotation of the foot than to position the ankle in the appropriate degree of dorsiflexion.[29,35]

If the possibility of subtle instability is uncertain, live fluoroscopic analysis of the ankle can also be performed. This may be completed preoperatively if the patient tolerates it or intraoperatively after fracture stabilization.[21] Stress maneuvers under fluoroscopy should include both eversion and lateral translation, as well as external rotation. Femino and colleagues[27] performed a biomechanical cadaveric analysis and advocated that, during external rotation stress, the foot to be in a varus position to lock out the hindfoot and midfoot. They found varus positioning of the foot during external rotation was more effective than the valgus position for displacement stress testing of the deltoid and syndesmosis (**Fig. 4**).

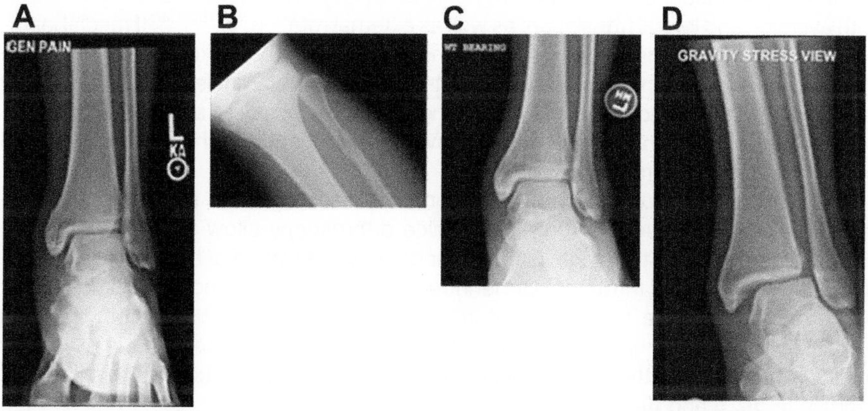

Fig. 4. (*A*) Nonweightbearing radiograph shows no signs of instability. (*B*) Proximal tibia-fibula radiograph shows proximal fibula fracture, indicating potential instability of the ankle. (*C*) Weightbearing radiograph of the ankle. There is still no sign of instability. (*D*) Gravity stress views of the ankle unmask instability of both the medial deltoid and distal tibiofibular syndesmosis.

MRI Versus Computed Tomography Scan

Advanced imaging, such as computed tomography (CT) or MRI, may be warranted in fractures that are not as clear-cut with a stressed radiograph. MRI is helpful in evaluating the extent of superficial versus deep deltoid involvement. Interestingly, MRI studies have shown that, with isolated fibula fractures, partial syndesmotic and/or deltoid tears are also identified in almost every case, even when the medial clear space is not widened. MRI also indicates whether an osteochondral lesion of the talus is also present. CT scans give insight into the extent of the osseous involvement. CT is also an effective tool for evaluating subtle syndesmotic injuries and malrotations of the fracture fragments.[36–38]

TREATMENT

Conservative Treatment

Nondisplaced ankle fractures suspicious for syndesmotic or deltoid injury should be evaluated with stress imaging. If all radiographic parameters remain within normal limits and the ankle is deemed stable, patients may be treated with periods of no weightbearing and immobilization. If osseous or soft tissue instability or displacement is identified, surgical treatment should be considered on a case-by-case basis, considering the patients comorbidities, physical demands, and activity level.

Surgical Treatment: When to Repair

The decision for ankle fracture surgical repair is often determined by the fracture features such as location, displacement, and pattern. For obvious deltoid injuries, such as extreme widening of the medial clear space, the decision to repair the deltoid can be assumed preoperatively. However, with subtle deltoid injuries, fractures around the ankle should be repaired via standard AO (Arbeitsgemeinschaft für Osteosynthesefragen) techniques, following which the soft tissues may then be assessed.[13,14,21,39] There is some debate regarding whether to repair the deltoid or the syndesmosis first. Both maintain critical roles in mortise stability. Typically, the syndesmosis is evaluated via intraoperative fluoroscopy and stress maneuvers after the fractures have been fixated. Following syndesmotic assessment and fixation, if necessary, the deltoid is evaluated. Static images should be compared with stress images. The ankle should be stressed with eversion and lateral translation, as well as external rotation.[13–15,21,40] If medial instability is encountered, the surgeon should consider primary repair of the deltoid to restore stability to the medial ankle. Unfortunately, stressing the medial ankle after fracture repair is often a neglected technique. Incorporating deltoid assessment and repair, if necessary, as part of ankle fracture treatment provides the patient with the highest likelihood of a satisfactory outcome.

Ankle arthroscopy in ankle fractures is an excellent diagnostic tool to evaluate the injury to the soft tissue. Not only does ankle arthroscopy allow for decompression of the hemarthrosis of the ankle, it allows for direct visualization of the deltoid and syndesmotic ligaments.[40] Intraarticular debridement of the deltoid and syndesmosis may aid in reduction of the complex fracture. More often than not, the deltoid ligament avulses off the distal tibia and invaginates into the medial gutter. This may hinder the initial reduction of the distal fibula fracture and overall restoration of the ankle joint mortise (**Figs. 5** and **6**).

HOW TO REPAIR

If medial instability is identified, surgical reconstruction should be considered. There is debate about whether to fixate the syndesmosis before fixing the deltoid

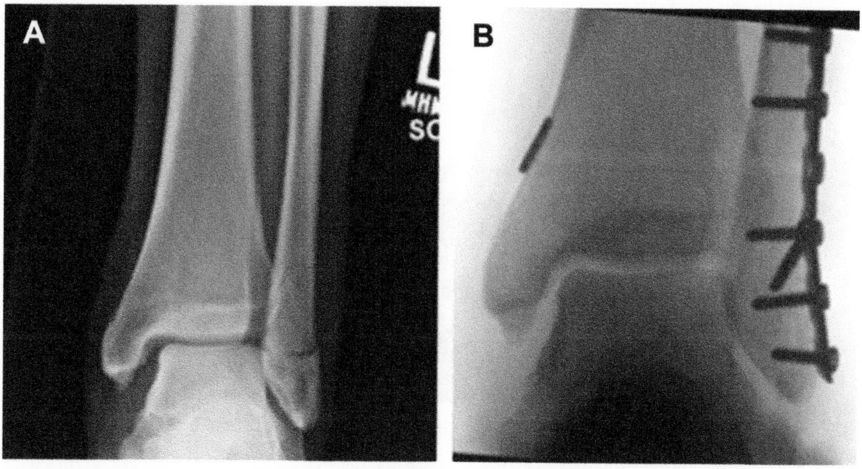

Fig. 5. (*A*) Fibula fracture with signs of medial deltoid instability. (*B*) Intraoperative stress maneuvers after fibula and syndesmosis fixation shows no signs of deltoid instability. Negative stress images indicate stable ankle has been achieved and no deltoid repair is necessary for this patient.

or vice versa. The authors suggest standard open reduction and internal fixation of the fibula fracture, followed by debridement and repair of the deltoid. In certain scenarios an insufficient deltoid may present as syndesmotic instability although, anatomically, this is not the case. The authors recommend an open repair with placement of anchors in the distal tibia. Advancement of the deep deltoid ligament is then performed. The superficial deltoid can then be reconstructed with either another suture anchor or suture to the periosteum. If continued widening persists, the addition of syndesmotic fixation can be added to offload the deltoid repair (**Figs. 7** and **8**).

In the case of true syndesmotic instability with a deltoid injury, the authors suggest open reduction and internal fixation of fibula; preparation for repair of the deltoid ligament, with anchors; syndesmotic repair; and, finally, advancement with final

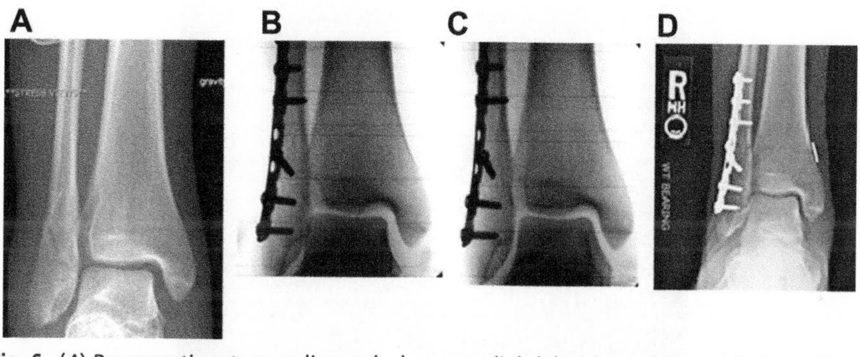

Fig. 6. (*A*) Preoperative stress radiograph shows medial deltoid instability with distal fibula fracture. (*B*) Intraoperative image shows signs of persistent medial deltoid instability. (*C*) Intraoperative stress image shows deltoid stability after primary repair. (*D*) Final weightbearing postoperative radiograph.

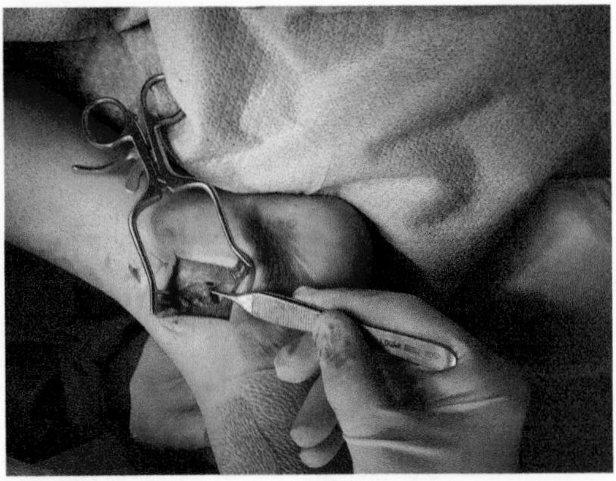

Fig. 7. Intraoperative close-up photograph demonstrates midsubstance tearing of the anterior portion of the deltoid.

tensioning of the deltoid. This technique allows for increased accuracy in reducing the syndesmosis and obtaining appropriate tension on the deltoid ligament reconstruction.

Open Primary Repair

There are several surgical approaches for management of a deltoid disruption. The approach depends on surgeon preference and comfort. The standard approach includes an incision over the distal aspect of the medial malleolus, curving slightly anterior and distal. This incision is superior to the course of the posterior tibial tendon. An anterior incision over the medial malleolus extending distally and posteriorly may also be used. Both surgical approaches will give the surgeon adequate visualization of partial-thickness and full-thickness tears of the anterior and middle portions of the deltoid ligament.

When the deltoid has avulsed from the medial malleolus, we prefer to use bone anchors for repair of this portion. The bone anchors are placed on the anterior and distal surfaces of the medial malleolus (**Fig. 9**). We prefer a number 2 suture with

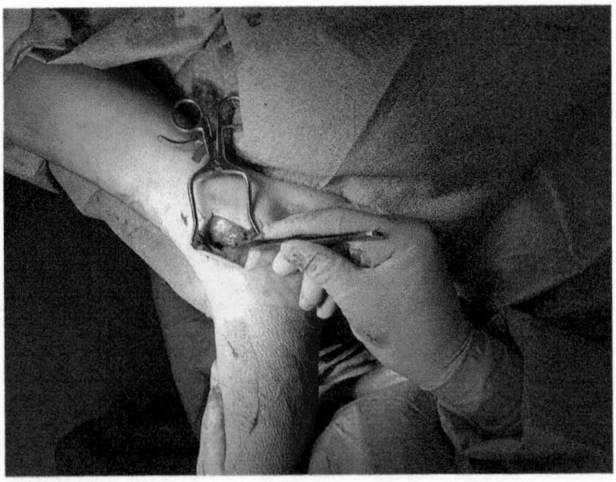

Fig. 8. Intraoperative distance photograph demonstrates midsubstance tearing of the anterior portion of the deltoid.

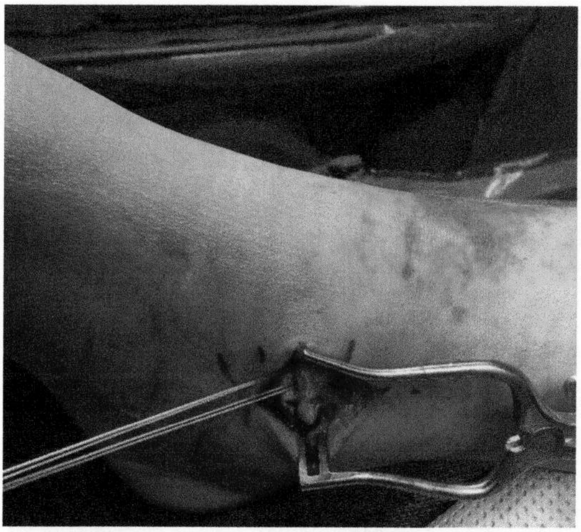

Fig. 9. Deltoid has avulsed from the medial malleolus with bone anchors for repair of this portion.

the anchors for this repair. Full-thickness suture passes into the deltoid are performed with each of the suture limbs. The ankle is then inverted and held in place while the sutures are tied appropriately. A third suture anchor maybe placed on the medial face of the medial malleolus to further advance the superficial fibers. Alternatively, advancement of the superficial fibers to the periosteum may also be performed. There may be a role for internal augmentation of deltoid tears using larger tape-like sutures with anchors. However, repair should not solely rely on this but be done in conjunction with primary ligament repair. We reserve this for complete disruption of the superficial and deep deltoid, larger patients, or those with tenuous ligament fibers remaining. Most deltoid tears we have encountered involve the anterior aspect of the superficial deltoid avulsing from the medial malleolus, which we have been repaired using bone anchors.

If a full-thickness deltoid injury with posterior involvement is noted, an incision is made along the course of the posterior tibial tendon at the level of the medial malleolus. The posterior medial neurovascular structures should be protected, especially in the setting of an acute ankle fracture with swelling and posttraumatic changes to the soft tissues. The posterior tibial tendon is inspected and retracted inferiorly. A variety of deltoid tears may be encountered. The deep fascia is opened and initial inspection for a midsubstance tear is performed. If encountered, direct primary repair using sutures is completed. If the deep deltoid is torn from the talus, bone anchors may be placed into the medial body of the talus and used to repair the deep portion. If there is preoperative suspicion for deep deltoid disruption, it is preferable to start medially because we have found it is easier to access this area while the ankle is unstable. However, before final tension of the ligament repair, we prefer to wait until all fractures have been reduced and fixated to avoid tensional changes in the soft tissues that may occur from fracture reduction. For example, if the deltoid is repaired and tensioned before a displaced fibula fracture is reduced, the medial deltoid repair will likely loosen as the length, translation, and rotation of the fibula is restored. If a deltoid ligament disruption occurs as a medial malleolus avulsion fracture, we recommend use of a hook plate for stabilization of the fracture fragment and advancement of the deltoid ligament.

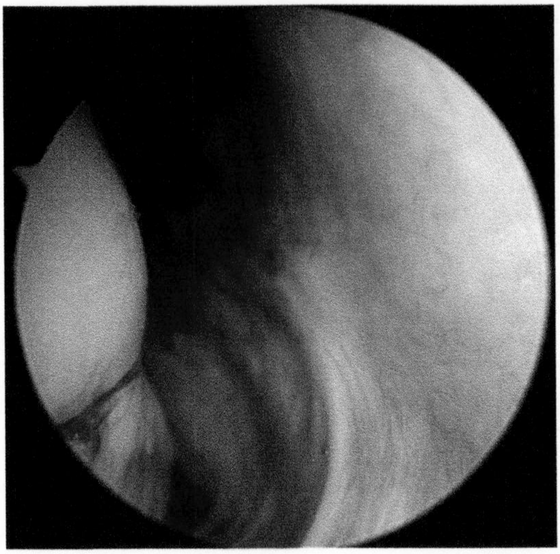

Fig. 10. Arthroscopic photograph demonstrates acute deltoid tear associated with ankle fracture.

Arthroscopic Repair

Patients with comorbidities increasing their risk for incisional complications or patients with anterior partial deltoid tears who demonstrate instability may benefit from an all-arthroscopic repair. This can be performed for deltoid tear with or without association of fractures around the ankle. Radiographs may not always accurately predict deltoid injuries, which is why some investigators have suggested arthroscopy as a means of further inspection and documentation of possible deltoid injuries.[17]

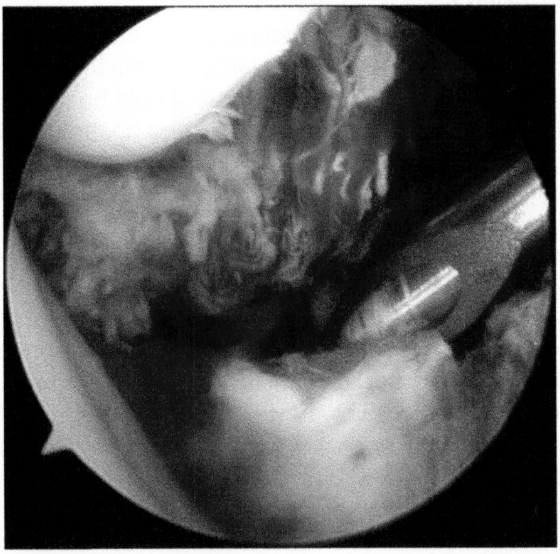

Fig. 11. Arthroscopic photograph demonstrates acute deltoid tear associated with ankle fracture.

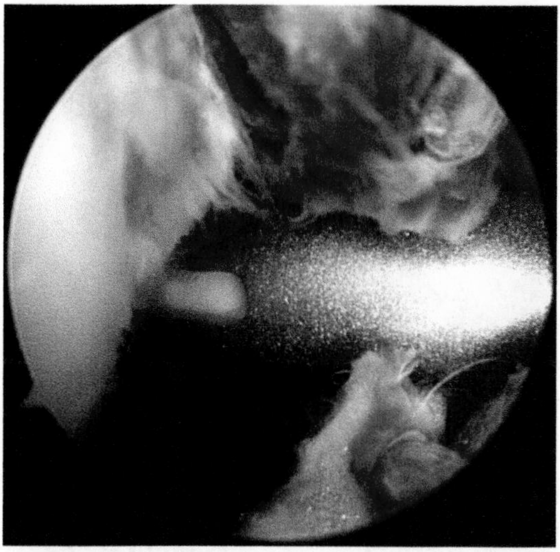

Fig. 12. Arthroscopic image of bone anchor placement in the medial malleolus.

If an arthroscopic assessment of the ankle is being performed before fracture stabilization and a deltoid tear is encountered that demonstrates instability, as discussed previously, the anchors and suture can be placed before fracture repair. Again, the final tension should be secured or hand tied after fracture repair, similar to the open approach, to avoid ligament tensional changes after fracture reduction.

Deltoid avulsion from the medial malleolus confirmed via arthroscopy is repairable via a minimally invasive arthroscopic technique. Midsubstance tearing or avulsion from the talus is more difficult via arthroscopic approach and is best repaired in an open fashion. One or 2 bone anchors may be placed into the medial malleolus

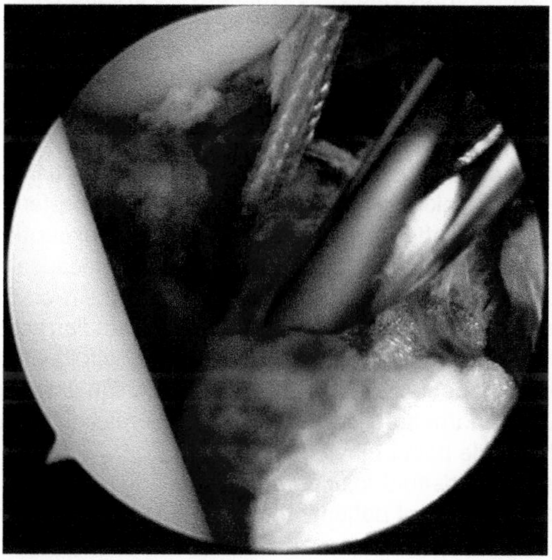

Fig. 13. Arthroscopic image using suture passer to capture and pass sutures through the deltoid arthroscopically.

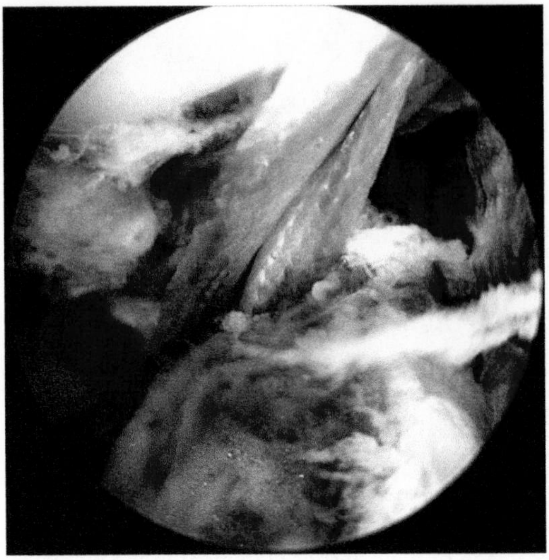

Fig. 14. Arthroscopic image demonstrates sutures placed to repair deltoid tear before final tensioning.

under arthroscopic guidance through the anteromedial portal. The associated anchor sutures then exit the portal. A suture passer device is then used to pass the sutures, as visualized via the arthroscope, through the deltoid and exiting medially through the skin. A small accessory incision is made just superior to the posterior tibial tendon to ensure the sutures avoid breeching this structure. When the anchors have been placed, the sutures adequately within the deltoid, and associated fractures have been repaired, the ankle is then held in a neutral dorsiflexion with slight inversion and the sutures are hand tied or an arthroscopic knot pusher is used to repair the torn portion of the deltoid back into good apposition and tension with the medial malleolus. Fluoroscopic stress maneuvers are then performed to confirm adequate repair. If instability persists, conversion to an open approach is then indicated (**Figs. 10–14**).

SUMMARY

A consensus has not yet been achieved regarding repairing partial or complete deltoid rupture associated with ankle fractures. It is the authors' preference to perform a repair if instability persists after fracture stabilization. The exception to this involves an obvious frank complete tear with significant disruption because we find it is easier to repair the deltoid before fracture stabilization and then tension the repair after the fractures are fixated. Given the paucity of high-powered studies arguing for or against repair, we choose to maintain a low threshold for medial deltoid inspection and repair. We think the ability to inspect the medial aspect of the joint, allowing for treatment of osteochondral injuries and/or soft tissue disruption, decreases the number of patients with residual medial ankle pain or instability.

Some studies suggest deltoid injuries heal uneventfully without repair. However, other studies report a subset of patients that continues to present with medial gutter pain and instability. This raises the question of whether those patients would have had improved outcome with a primary repair.[4,7–10] Ultimately, the question each surgeon must answer is: does the risk of complications from a medial incision, as well as the increased surgical time and expense, justify attempts at improving outcomes for such patients? It should be remembered that chronic instability of the tibiotalar joint leads to abnormal mechanics and degradation of the joint. Horisberger and colleagues[14] noted a 20.4% incidence of posttraumatic ankle osteoarthritis in patients with an untreated deltoid ligament injury.

In the authors' experience, the benefits of deltoid repair include the potential for earlier weightbearing with less fear of deltoid laxity developing. As one of the most vital structures of ankle instability, the argument for restoring the overall continuity, length, and tension is quite strong. Creating a medial incision, if soft tissues allow, is certainly justifiable if surgeons think instability persists. As the circumstances that warrant deltoid repair are better understood, and these parameters continue to be defined, it is imperative that surgeons confirm if the medial ankle complex is sufficient and stable for each patient. The authors advocate that chronic medial ankle pathologic conditions are often difficult to treat and all attempts should be made in an effort to minimize these negative outcomes. Ultimately, each surgeon should make the decision to repair the deltoid ligament on a case-by-case basis.

REFERENCES

1. Campbell K, Michalski M, Wilson K, et al. The ligament anatomy of the deltoid complex of the ankle: a qualitative and quantitative anatomical study. J Bone Joint Surg Am 2014;96(8):e62.
2. Panchani P, Chappell T, Moore G, et al. Anatomic study of the deltoid ligament of the ankle. Foot Ankle Int 2014;35(9):916–21.
3. Baird R, Jackson S. Fractures of the distal part of the fibula with associated disruption of the deltoid ligament. Treatment without repair of the deltoid ligament. J Bone Joint Surg Am 1987;69(9):1346–52.
4. Zeegers A, van der Werken C. Rupture of the deltoid ligament in ankle fractures: should it be repaired? Injury 1989;20(1):39–41.
5. Heim U. Die Verletzungen des medialen Bandapparates am oberen Sprunggelenk und ihre Behandlung. Hefte Unfallheilkd 1978;(131):125–6.
6. De Souza L, Gustilo R, Meyer T. Results of operative treatment of displaced external rotation-abduction fractures of the ankle. J Bone Joint Surg Am 1985; 67(7):1066–74.
7. Harper M. The deltoid ligament. An evaluation of need for surgical repair. Clin Orthop Relat Res 1988;(226):156–68.
8. Johnson D, Hill J. Fracture-dislocation of the ankle with rupture of the deltoid ligament. Injury 1988;19(2):59–61.
9. Stufkens S, van den Bekerom M, Knupp M, et al. The diagnosis and treatment of deltoid ligament lesions in supination-external rotation ankle fractures: a review. Strategies Trauma Limb Reconstr 2012;7(2):73–85.
10. Strömsöe K, Höqevold HE, Skjeldal S, et al. The repair of a ruptured deltoid ligament is not necessary in ankle fractures. J Bone Joint Surg Br 1995;77(6):920–1.
11. Lee T, Jang K, Choi G, et al. The contribution of anterior deltoid ligament to ankle stability in isolated lateral malleolar fractures. Injury 2016;47(7):1581–5.
12. Hintermann B, Knupp M, Pagenstert G. Deltoid ligament injuries: diagnosis and management. Foot Ankle Clin 2006;11(3):625–37.
13. Lötscher P, Lang T, Zwicky L, et al. Osteoligamentous injuries of the medial ankle joint. Eur J Trauma Emerg Surg 2015;41(6):615–21.
14. Horisberger M, Valderrabano V, Hintermann B. Posttraumatic ankle osteoarthritis after ankle-related fractures. J Orthop Trauma 2009;23(1):60–7.

15. Tornetta P. Competence of the deltoid ligament in bimalleolar ankle fractures after medial malleolar fixation. J Bone Joint Surg Am 2000;82(6):843–8.
16. Schuberth J, Collman D, Rush S, et al. Deltoid ligament integrity in lateral malleolar fractures: a comparative analysis of arthroscopic and radiographic assessments. J Foot Ankle Surg 2004;43(1):20–9.
17. Kusnezov N, Eisenstein E, Diab N, et al. Medial malleolar fractures and associated deltoid ligament disruptions: current management controversies. Orthopedics 2017;40(2):e216–22.
18. Zhang T, Wan C, Ma B, et al. Case-control study on two suturing methods for the repairing of complete rupture of the deltoid ligament. Zhongguo Gu Shang 2016;29(5):408–14.
19. Hsu A, Anderson R. Foot and ankle injuries in American football. Am J Orthop 2016;45(6):358–67.
20. Yu G, Zhang M, Aiyer A, et al. Repair of the acute deltoid ligament complex rupture associated with ankle fractures: a multicenter clinical study. J Foot Ankle Surg 2015;54(2):198–202.
21. Wang X, Zhang C, Yin J, et al. Treatment of medial malleolus or pure deltoid ligament injury in patients with supination-external rotation type IV ankle fractures. Orthop Surg 2017;9(1):42–8.
22. Bauer M, Bergström B, Hemborg A, et al. Malleolar fractures: nonoperative versus operative treatment. A controlled study. Clin Orthop Relat Res 1985;199:17–27.
23. Lindsjö U. Operative treatment of ankle fracture-dislocations. A follow-up study of 306/321 consecutive cases. Clin Orthop Relat Res 1985;199:28–38.
24. Pettrone F, Gail M, Pee D, et al. Quantitative criteria for prediction of the results after displaced fracture of the ankle. J Bone Joint Surg Am 1983;65A:667–77.
25. Yde J, Kristensen KD. Ankle fractures: supination-eversion fractures of stage IV. Primary and late results of operative and non-operative treatment. Acta Orthop Scand 1980;51:981–90.
26. Femino JE, Vaseenon T, Phisitkul P, et al. Varus external rotation stress test for radiographic detection of deep deltoid ligament disruption with and without syndesmotic disruption: a cadaveric study. Foot Ankle Int 2013;34(2):251–60.
27. Hastie G, Akhtar S, Butt U, et al. Weightbearing radiograph facilitate functional treatment of ankle fractures of uncertain stability. J Foot Ankle Surg 2015;54(6):1042–6.
28. Boffeli T, Collier R, Gervais S. Two-view gravity stress imaging protocol for nondisplaced type II supination external rotation ankle fractures: introducing the gravity stress cross-table lateral view. J Foot Ankle Surg 2017;56(4):898–904.
29. LeBa T, Gugala Z, Morris R, et al. Gravity versus manual external rotation stress view in evaluating ankle stability: a prospective study. Foot Ankle Spec 2015;8(3):175–9.
30. Schock H, Pinzur M, Manion L, et al. The use of gravity or manual-stress radiograph in the assessment of supination-external rotation fractures of the ankle. J Bone Joint Surg Br 2007;89(8):1055–9.
31. Michelson J, Varner K, Checcone M. Diagnosing deltoid injury in ankle fractures: the gravity stress view. Clin Orthop Relat Res 2001;387:178–82.
32. Michelson J, Ahn U, Helgemo S. Motion of the ankle in a simulated supination-external rotation fracture model. J Bone Joint Surg Am 1996;78:1024–31.
33. Gill JB, Risko T, Raducan V, et al. Comparison of manual and gravity stress radiograph for the evaluation of supination-external rotation fibular fractures. J Bone Joint Surg Am 2007;89(5):994–9.

34. van den Bekerom M, Mutsaerts E, van Dijk C. Evaluation of the integrity of the deltoid ligament in supination external rotation ankle fractures: a systematic review of the literature. Arch Orthop Trauma Surg 2009;129(2):227–35.
35. Cheung Y, Perrich KD, Gui J, et al. MRI of isolated distal fibular fractures with widened medial clear space on stressed radiograph: which ligaments are interrupted? AJR Am J Roentgenol 2009;192(1):W7–12.
36. Jeong M, Choi Y, Kim Y, et al. Deltoid ligament in acute ankle injury: MR imaging analysis. Skeletal Radiol 2014;43(5):655–63.
37. Hermans J, Wentink N, Beumer A, et al. Correlation between radiological assessment of acute ankle fractures and syndesmotic injury on MRI. Skeletal Radiol 2012;41(7):787–801.
38. Lack W, Phisitkul P, Femino J. Anatomic deltoid ligament repair with anchor-to-post suture reinforcement: technique tip. Iowa Orthop J 2012;32:227–30.
39. Boss A, Hintermann B. Anatomical study of the medial ankle ligament complex. Foot Ankle Int 2002;23(6):547–53.
40. Schairer W, Nwachukwu B, Dare DM, et al. Arthroscopically assisted open reduction-internal fixation of ankle fractures: significance of the arthroscopic ankle drive-through sign. Arthrosc Tech 2016;5(2):e407–12.

Arthroscopic-Assisted Open Reduction Internal Fixation

Graham A. Hamilton, DPM[a,*],
Matthew D. Doyle, DPM, MS[b,c],
Francesca M. Castellucci-Garza, DPM, MS[b,c]

KEYWORDS

• Ankle • Arthroscopy • Fracture • Fracture fixation • Fracture reduction • Trauma

KEY POINTS

- Arthroscopy is a valuable tool to assist in fracture reduction and fixation by permitting direct visualization of the articular surface in addition to preserving the soft tissues.
- Standard ankle and subtalar portals for delivery of the instrumentation through the surgical wound are the most commonly used approaches. Gravity inflow for visualization and a high-speed shaver for preliminary debridement are key steps to allow for intra-articular fracture assessment.
- Intraoperative arthroscopy should always be used in conjunction with fluoroscopy to achieve reduction and assess implant placement.
- Reduction is achieved with reduction clamps, K-wires, or both.
- Arthroscopic technique is largely surgeon dependent. A surgeon should be comfortable with arthroscopy and techniques for fracture fixation and stabilization. This is not recommended for the novice arthroscopist.

INTRODUCTION

The term "arthroscopy" was first coined by Nordentoft in 1912.[1] Joint arthroscopy was then introduced in 1918 with a cadaveric knee joint by Takagi using a cystoscope.[2] In 1931, Burman attempted to insert an arthroscope in a cadaveric ankle. After his attempts, he concluded that the ankle joint was unfit for arthroscopy.[3] Later, Watanabe, a protégé of Takagi, furthered intrigue with newer devices and the concept of triangulation.[1,4] As instrumentation improved over the years, the interest in arthroscopy

Disclosure: The authors have nothing to disclose.
[a] Foot and Ankle Surgery, Department of Podiatric Surgery, Palo Alto Foundation Medical Group, 4000 Dublin Boulevard, Dublin, CA 94568, USA; [b] Department of Orthopedics, Kaiser San Francisco Bay Area Foot and Ankle Residency Program, Kaiser Permanente Oakland Medical Center, 275 West MacArthur Boulevard, Oakland, CA 94611, USA; [c] Department of Podiatry, Kaiser San Francisco Bay Area Foot and Ankle Residency Program, Kaiser Permanente Oakland Medical Center, 275 West MacArthur Boulevard, Oakland, CA 94611, USA
* Corresponding author.
E-mail address: Graham_hamilton@mac.com

Clin Podiatr Med Surg 35 (2018) 199–221
https://doi.org/10.1016/j.cpm.2017.12.004
0891-8422/18/

gained steam. The first reports of arthroscopy in the ankle were in the 1980s, followed by subtalar arthroscopy in 1985.[5–8] Its use has expanded in the body and is well documented throughout the biomedical literature.[9] Arthroscopy has now been used for many years in the foot and ankle, to diagnose and treat many conditions. Its role has also evolved over time and continues to expand. Current accepted uses for arthroscopy in the foot and ankle include osteochondral defects, synovitis, arthrofibrosis, soft tissue and osseous impingement, osteophytosis, and arthrodesis.[10–12] More recently, the application of arthroscopy in the foot and ankle has been used in acute trauma, to aid in the reduction of intra-articular fractures, as well as to visualize and potentially treat posttraumatic articular defects.[13–17] Traditionally, treatment of displaced, intra-articular fractures of the foot and ankle has required open techniques, where the fragments are reduced and internal fixation is delivered. Large surgical approaches do however carry risk. They can potentially disrupt the osseous blood supply and in turn hinder or delay fracture healing. These larger surgical exposures also have higher risks of wound complications, infection, delayed union, and nonunion. Smaller incisional approaches and the decreased overall morbidity associated with them have led to an expanded role for arthroscopy in the foot and ankle. Arthroscopic-assisted open reduction internal fixation (AA-ORIF), or arthroscopic reduction internal fixation, provides an added tool with low complication rates and may lead to earlier patient mobilization.[18] This technique also allows for direct visualization of the articular surface with the associated fracture lines and provides the surgeon the opportunity to gain precise reduction through a minimal soft tissue window.

Indications for Arthroscopic-Assisted Open Reduction Internal Fixation

- Ankle fractures: Weber type A fibula fractures, Weber type C fibula fractures, medial malleolus fractures, displaced bimalleolar and trimalleolar ankle fractures
- Pilon fractures
- Talus fracture
- Calcaneal fractures
- Tillaux fractures
- Triplane fractures

Contraindications for Arthroscopic-Assisted Open Reduction Internal Fixation

- Grossly contaminated or infected soft tissue
- Severe comminution requiring open reduction
- Severe joint arthritis
- Medical comorbidities making surgery unsafe

PATIENT WORKUP

Initial patient workup includes a physical examination and appropriate imaging of the extremity. Frequently, 3 views of the foot and ankle and 2 views of the leg are required for full examination. A thorough history should be obtained regarding any pertinent fracture mechanics. Closed reduction of any fracture or dislocation is performed expeditiously, and a well-padded splint is placed to the injured extremity. There are two windows to surgically fix the injury: the early and late periods. The early period is within 6 hours of the injury, whereas the late period is typically between days 6 and 12 after injury, once the soft tissue edema has settled. Incising the injured area between these two periods may increase the likelihood of wound problems. Certain fracture patterns require advanced imaging, such as computed tomography (CT), for a more thorough evaluation of the injury and to assist in surgical planning. A CT scan is commonly indicated in Pilon, triplane, Tillaux, Salter-Harris, calcaneus, talus, and certain ankle fractures.

ARTHROSCOPIC TECHNIQUE

The technique may be achieved using large (4.0-mm) or small joint (2.7-mm) and 30° or 70° arthroscopes. Selection of the arthroscope size depends on the size of the patient and the joint being explored. Standard anteromedial and anterolateral ankle portals can be used for almost all fracture patterns. Sometimes visualization necessitates an accessory anteromedial or anterolateral portal. In certain fractures, subtalar arthroscopy is used with standard stacked anterolateral portals and potentially a posterolateral portal. The authors recommend avoiding arthroscopic pumps with these fracture cases and prefer gravity inflow. To assist with distention visualization, a separate inflow and outflow portal can be used with 3- to 4-L bags of lactated ringer's solution. It is recommended to hang the solution 3 feet above the table. In most cases, distraction is not required to enter the joint. On occasion, it is needed to enter and fully access the entire ankle joint. The Kerlex roll technique can be used for manual distraction if necessary[19]. The authors recommend a modification to this technique using noninvasive straps, which is technically easier to perform (**Fig. 1**). Upon first entering the joint, the surgeon typically encounters debris and hematoma, which can be evacuated with a high-speed shaver, so the fracture lines can be appreciated. Impacted fragments that are determined to be too small to fix can be removed. Once the fracture is visible, adequate reduction, stabilization, and fixation can be achieved.

ANKLE FRACTURES

Ankle fractures in adults that are displaced and unstable have traditionally shown favorable results with standard open reduction and stabilization with internal fixation.[20–24] Occasionally, results may be unsatisfactory even in the presence of anatomic reduction.[25–27] Some fracture types however lend themselves well to the use of arthroscopically assisted minimally invasive techniques. Arthroscopy allows the surgeon to directly visualize the fracture reduction, identify concomitant abnormality, or primarily treat articular defects. It also provides minimal disruption to the soft tissue envelope as compared with an open approach. Ankle fractures that are most amenable to arthroscopic-assisted reduction and fixation include isolated lateral or

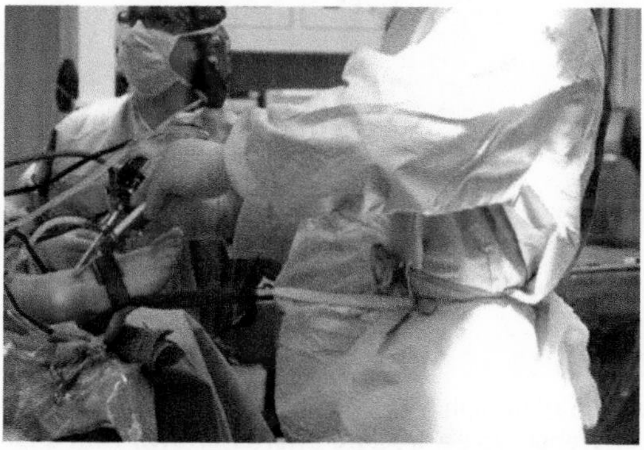

Fig. 1. Noninvasive distraction with a Kerlex roll and commercially available ankle strap.

medial malleolar fractures that are not significantly displaced, fractures of the proximal fibula with syndesmotic disruption, as well as certain mildly displaced bimalleolar or trimalleolar fractures.

The isolated transverse fracture of the lateral malleolus below the level of the distal syndesmosis, Weber A type, is typically gapped or slightly displaced laterally but is usually not significantly displaced (**Fig. 2**). This fracture line can easily be visualized arthroscopically via use of an anteromedial portal. The use of a 70°arthroscope is usually very beneficial to see the inferior portions of the lateral gutter of the ankle. Reduction can be achieved either via manual external pressure or with a probe intra-articularly. Alternatively, the fracture can be manipulated and reduced percutaneously with pointed reduction forceps (**Fig. 3**). Once reduced and temporarily stabilized, reduction is visualized arthroscopically and confirmed with the image intensifier (**Fig. 4**). Fixation is achieved with a percutaneous cannulated intramedullary lag screw, which is delivered from the tip of the lateral malleolus aiming proximally and advanced into the fibular shaft (**Fig. 5**).

Medial malleolus fractures, particularly isolated oblique or vertically oriented fractures, can be reduced and fixated in a similar arthroscopic manner to isolated, transverse infrasyndesmotic fibular fractures (**Fig. 6**). The fracture is arthroscopically visualized at the medial bend of the tibia with the arthroscope in the anterolateral portal. The anteromedial portal is used for fracture debridement and manipulation. After appropriate anatomic reduction, fixation of the oblique type fracture can be achieved with 2 cannulated lag screws (**Fig. 7**). The more vertically oriented "shear type" fracture usually requires stabilization with a percutaneously placed antiglide plate in order to neutralize the shear forces. Periosteal interposition may prevent anatomic reduction, thus necessitating formal ORIF, or in some situations, a small incision at the apex of the fracture can aid in reduction. It is important to identify that many vertically

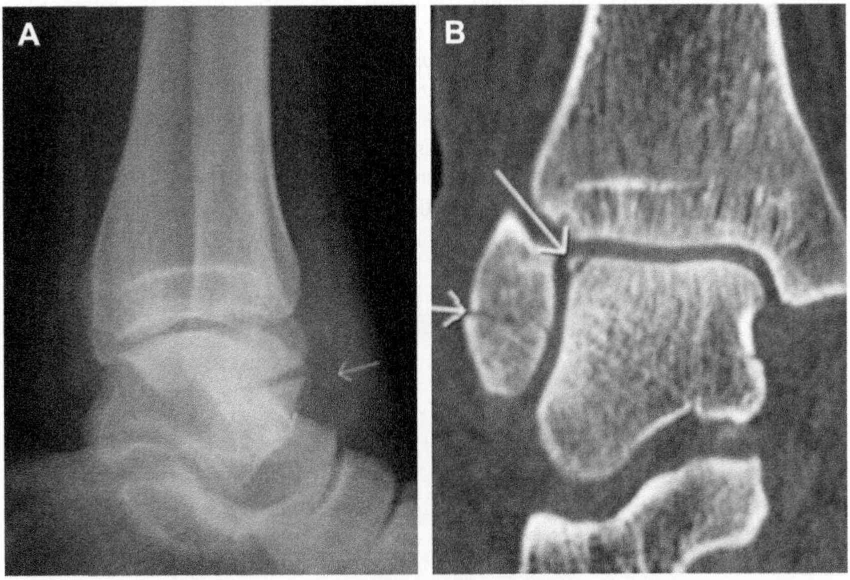

Fig. 2. (*A*) Lateral ankle radiograph. Arrow demonstrates gapping of the distal fibula fracture. (*B*) CT image of Weber type A fracture (*shorter arrow*), with a lateral osteochondral lesion of the talus (*longer arrow*).

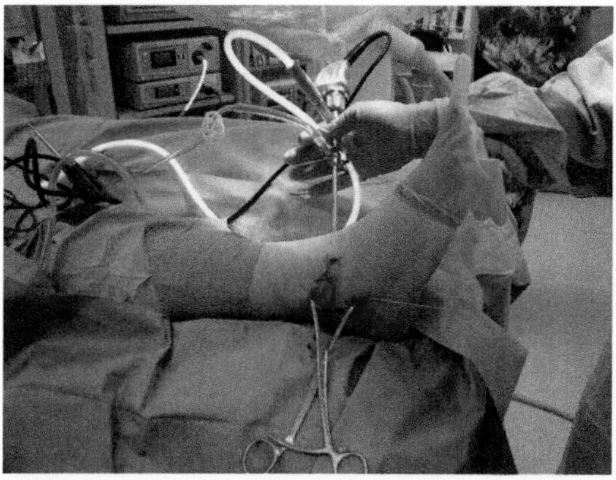

Fig. 3. Demonstration of percutaneous reduction of a gapped Weber type A fibula fracture.

oriented medial malleolar fractures have concomitant osteochondral injuries of the medial talar shoulder or impaction of the tibial plafond. One could attempt to arthroscopically disimpact the fragments, although this situation typically commands traditional open methods. The transverse fracture of the medial malleolus is usually more resistant to the arthroscopic-assisted technique secondary to periosteal incarceration at the fracture margins. In addition, the transverse orientation of the fracture makes it problematic to reduce percutaneously with reduction forceps.

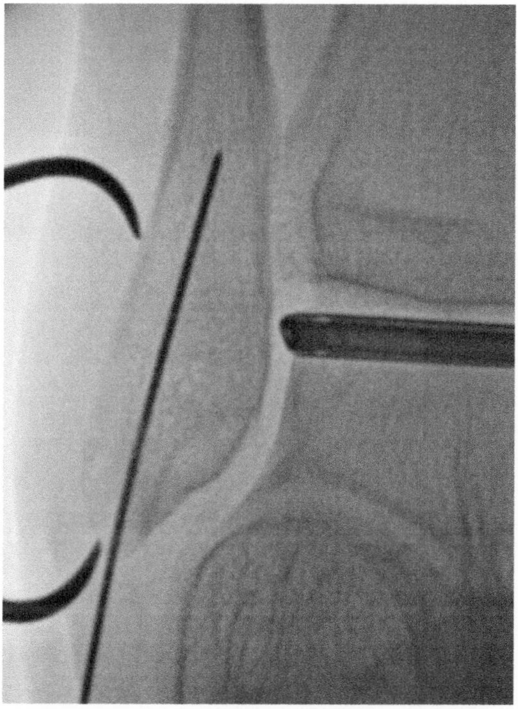

Fig. 4. Fluoroscopic confirmation of a percutaneously reduced distal fibula fracture with temporary stabilization.

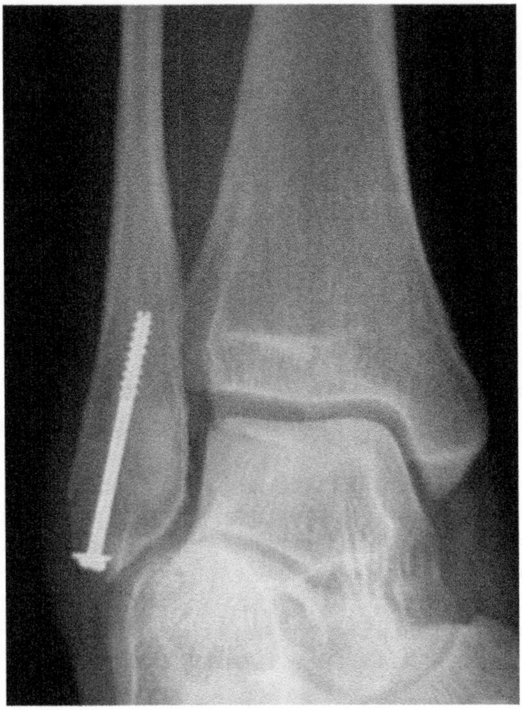

Fig. 5. Cannulated lag screw compressing the distal fibula.

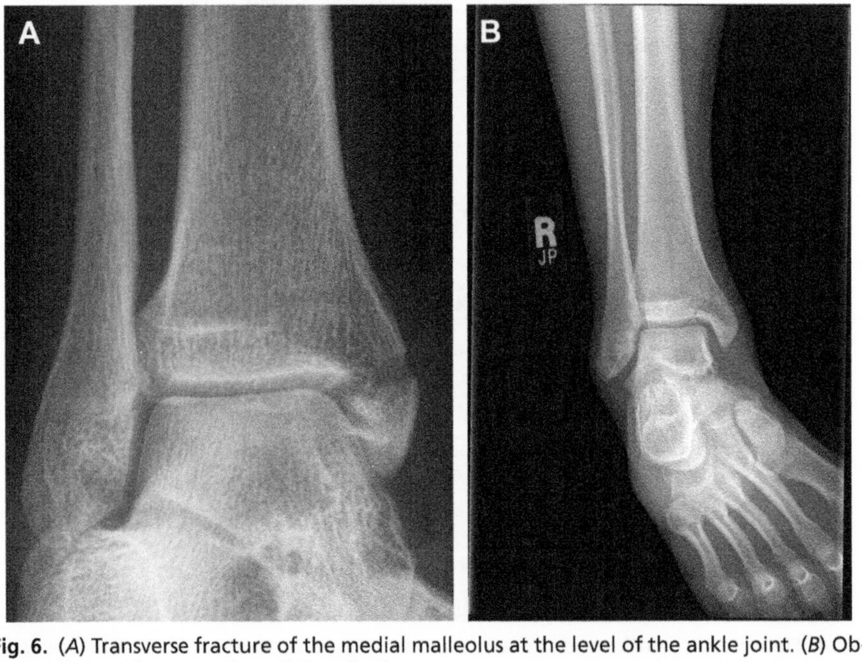

Fig. 6. (*A*) Transverse fracture of the medial malleolus at the level of the ankle joint. (*B*) Oblique oriented fracture of medial malleolus.

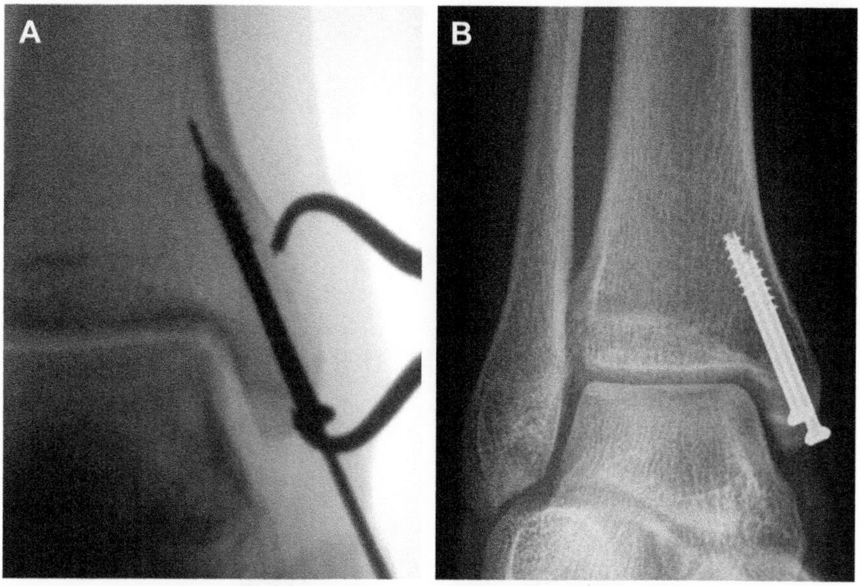

Fig. 7. (*A*) Percutaneous reduction of the medial malleolus and visualization under fluoroscopy. (*B*) Anatomic alignment postpercutaneous reduction and fixation.

Proximal fibula fractures (Maisonneuve), Weber type C, are yet another injury that can be treated through an arthroscopically assisted approach.[28] The proximal fibula fracture is usually minimally displaced and is fixated in an indirect manner. In these injuries, arthroscopic evaluation of the tibiofibular relationship may lead to improved accuracy of syndesmotic reduction given the high percentage of malreduction in the traditional open approach.[29] Once reduced, the syndesmosis can be provisionally stabilized and syndesmotic screws can be delivered percutaneously with fluoroscopic assistance. An unstable syndesmotic (high ankle sprain) injury can also be managed in the same manner.

Minimally displaced bimalleolar or trimalleolar fractures under certain circumstances can be treated with arthroscopically assisted minimally invasive techniques (**Fig. 8**). The arthroscope can be inserted initially through the traditional ankle portals, or it can be placed through an open arthrotomy incision. The arthroscope can aid in reduction and in identifying and potentially treating any articular damage. It may be necessary to perform traditional ORIF on one side and fixate the other side in minimally invasive technique with the fracture pattern as a guide.

The bimalleolar equivalent fracture is a unique pattern with a fracture of the fibula along with deltoid disruption (**Fig. 9**). Arthroscopic assistance is quite useful for this fracture pattern. The fibula fracture should be anatomically reduced and fixated either via traditional ORIF or through a minimally invasive technique (**Fig. 10**). It is well known that the loss of deltoid integrity increases the instability of the ankle fracture.[29] However, if the fibula is anatomically reduced and fixated, and the syndesmosis is stable, the deltoid does not require primary repair. The arthroscope is used to evaluate any osteochondral damage, especially on the medial aspect of the talar dome.

Through more recent evidence, it appears there is a higher incidence of articular injury in ankle fractures than previously understood. Ferkel and Orwin[30] reported that approximately 80% of ankle fractures have a chondral or osteochondral lesion. In another study,

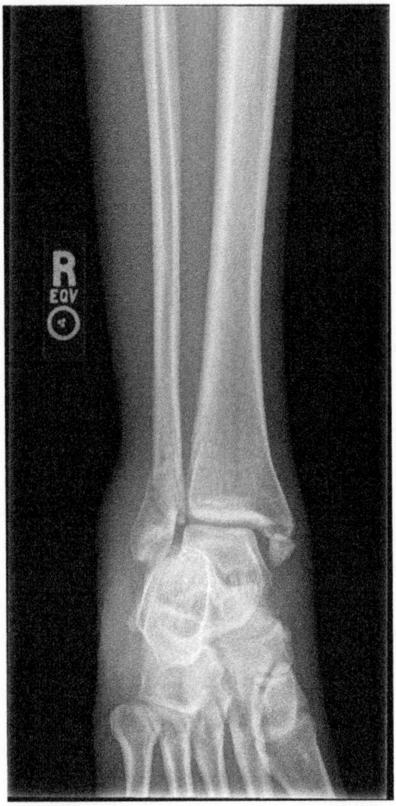

Fig. 8. Bimalleolar ankle fracture.

Leontaritis and colleagues[17] found that in 283 ankle fractures that underwent ORIF in addition to arthroscopy, 73% were observed to have chondral defects. Hintermann and colleagues[14] reported that frequency and severity of chondral injuries increased in Weber type C as compared with type B injuries, but did not increase between types B and A injuries. Ono and colleagues[16] determined that chondral lesions occurred in all fracture types, and there is no association between type of injury and chondral damage severity. They also concluded that fracture type did not correlate with the site of the chondral injury. The articular damage can range from impactions and excoriations to chondral or osteochondral fragments. Some postulate that occult chondral injury at the time of ankle fracture may lead to residual symptoms posttraumatically.[13] Thus, if one was to use arthroscopy, an osteochondral fragment could be excised, microfracture could be performed, or in the case of impactions/excoriations, they can be documented and used to assess the prognosis.

PILON FRACTURES

Pilon fractures are the result of high-energy injuries with axial compression and/or rotation involving the articular surface of the distal tibia (**Fig. 11**). They comprise between 1% and 10% of lower extremity fractures.[31,32] These injuries are damaging to the osseous and soft tissue structures, and over the years, a 2-staged protocol using an external fixator has been adopted to allow the soft tissue

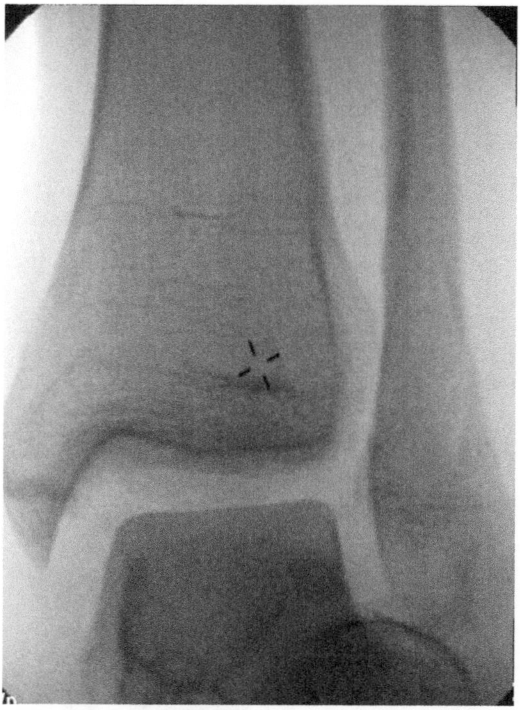

Fig. 9. Bimalleolar equivalent ankle fracture.

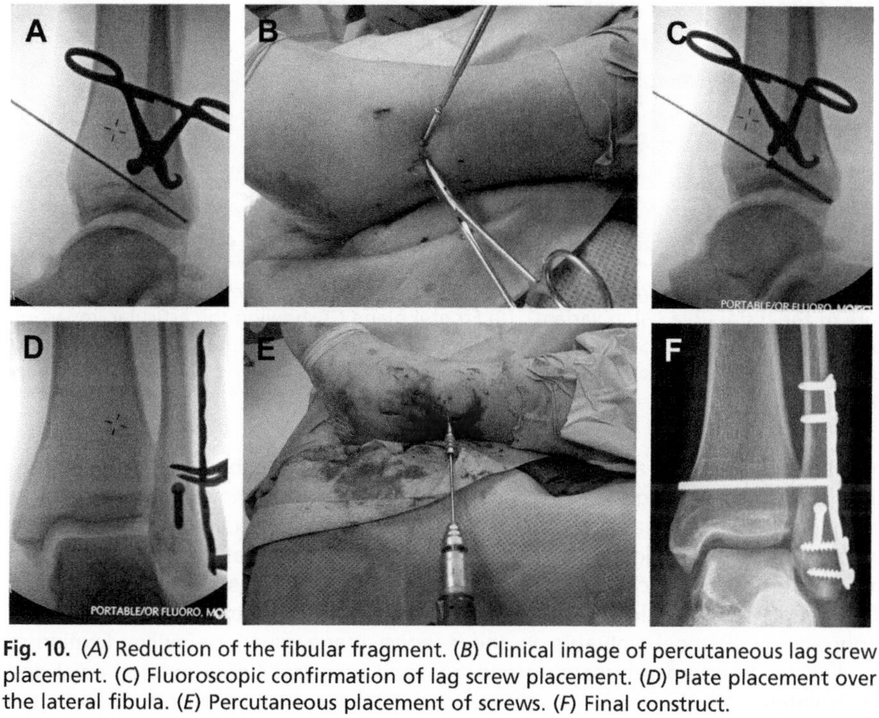

Fig. 10. (*A*) Reduction of the fibular fragment. (*B*) Clinical image of percutaneous lag screw placement. (*C*) Fluoroscopic confirmation of lag screw placement. (*D*) Plate placement over the lateral fibula. (*E*) Percutaneous placement of screws. (*F*) Final construct.

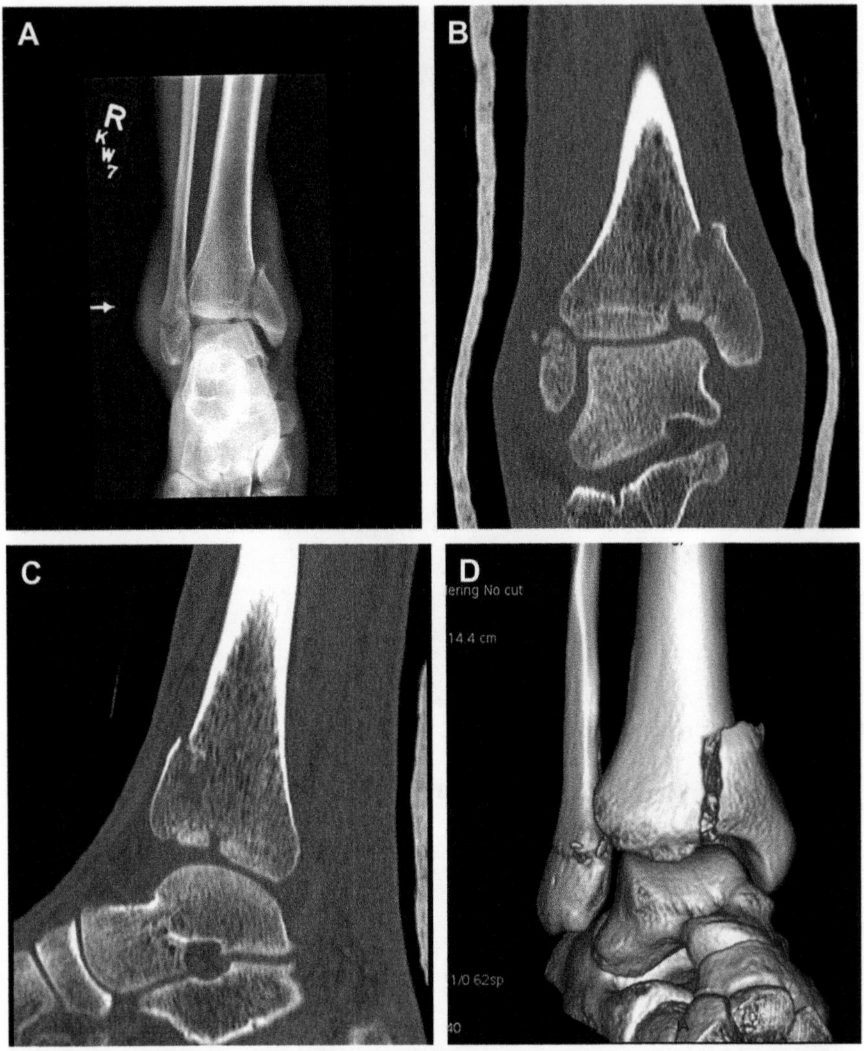

Fig. 11. (*A*) Anteroposterior (AP) radiograph of a Weber A fracture and medial shear fracture of the distal tibia (Pilon variant). (*B*) Frontal plane CT showing the articular impaction of the tibila plafond. (*C*) Sagittal plane CT demonstrating anterior displacement of the articular surface. (*D*) Three-dimensional (3D) reconstructed CT showing the complete injury pattern.

envelope to recover and decrease the rate of infection before definitive fixation.[33,34] Between stages, a CT is obtained for surgical planning (**Fig. 12**). At 10-years postinjury, a greater degree of arthritis occurs in open injuries with articular incongruity and malalignment.[35] Also, the greater severity of the fracture pattern has led to poorer clinical outcomes and quicker onset of posttraumatic arthritis.[36] Thus, quality of reduction plays a vital role in patient outcomes and quality of life.[37] Arthroscopy is most valuable in the second stage when definitive fixation is applied. A standard arthroscope can be used with traditional anteromedial and anterolateral ankle portals to assess the articular congruity and debride the

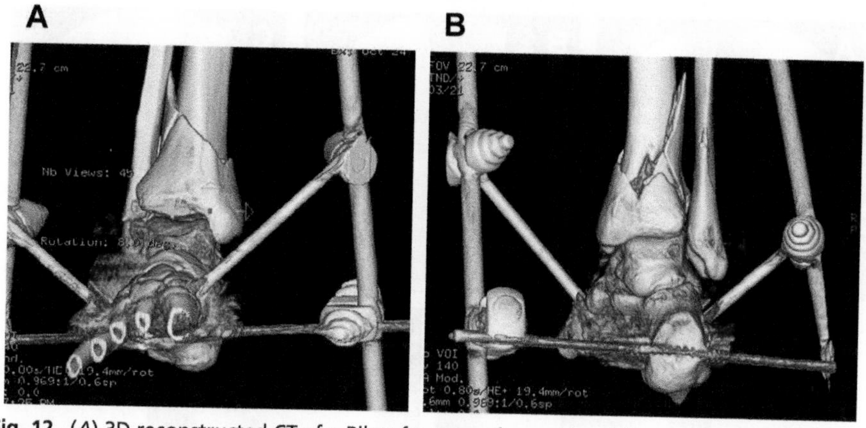

Fig. 12. (*A*) 3D reconstructed CT of a Pilon fracture after external fixator placement for pre-operative planning. (*B*) Posterior view of 3D CT.

articular surface and soft tissue, although it can also be placed directly into open incisions (**Fig. 13**). Placement directly into fracture fragments for reduction and evaluation of die-punch fragments is also a useful tool. Intraoperative fluoroscopy should be used before definitive fixation (**Fig. 14**). The literature consists of single

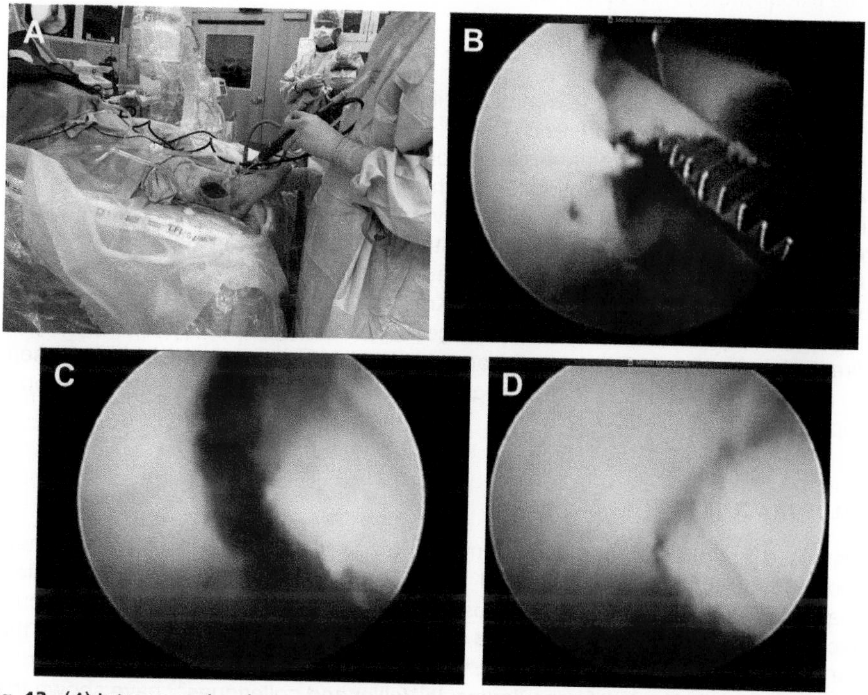

Fig. 13. (*A*) Intraoperative demonstration of arthroscopic evaluation using standard antero-medial and anterolateral ankle portals in a Pilon variant. (*B*) Arthroscopic debridement of a Pilon fracture removing incarcerated fragment and hematoma. (*C*) Arthroscopic evaluation of the central fracture line of the distal tibia after intercalary fragment removal. (*D*) Final fracture reduction of the distal tibial plafond.

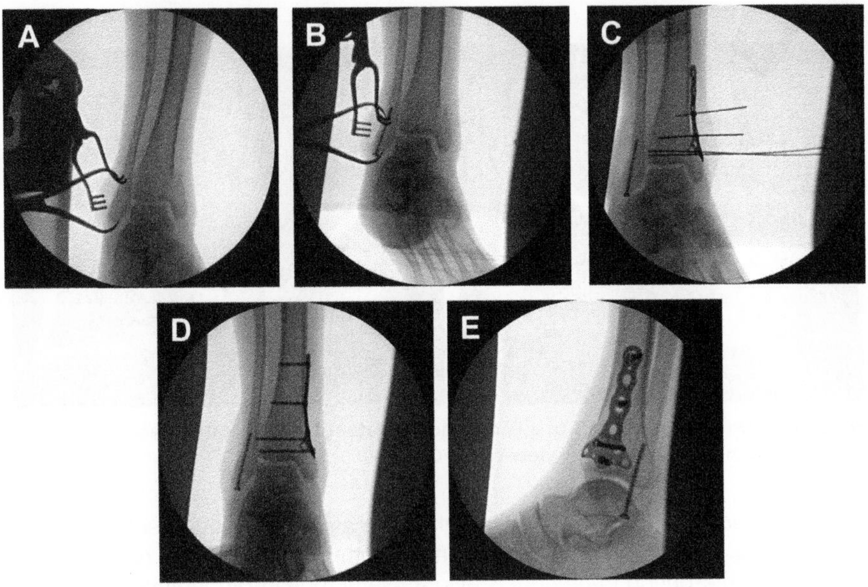

Fig. 14. (*A*) Initial reduction step. (*B*) Step 2. Fibular fracture fixation. (*C*) Temporary stabilization and medial plate insertion. (*D*) Fluoroscopic AP image of final reduction and hardware placement. (*E*) Final reduction.

case reports and small case series of Pilon fractures managed with arthroscopic assistance.[38–41] Hammond and Crist[38] described using the distal aspect of the lateral incision for the anterolateral portal along with a standard anteromedial portal. Arthroscopy was administered while the external fixator remained in place from the previous stage of surgery to prevent further need for distraction. Anatomic reduction is confirmed before definitive fixation. Salton and colleagues[40] used standard arthroscopic portals to assess reduction in a limited incision and percutaneous approach in 3 cases. Kralinger and colleagues[41] debrided the tibial articular surface with an arthroscope and stated that arthroscopy allows direct visualization of the joint surface. Its application seems to be most useful in assessing the ankle joint congruity during minimally invasive and open approaches.

TALUS FRACTURES

Displaced fractures of the talus are most often treated with ORIF. Most talar neck and body fractures are displaced and require open approaches to achieve anatomic reduction and minimize postoperative complications, such as avascular necrosis, posttraumatic arthritis, and angular deformity. It is well documented that the blood supply to the talus is poor.[42–44] Open approaches have also reported on the increased likelihood of vascular insult. Vallier and colleagues[45] have shown that open, comminuted fractures have a higher propensity for developing avascular necrosis. Traditional open reduction techniques require a combined medial and lateral longitudinal incision.[46,47] This approach offers the surgeon the clear benefit of direct fracture visualization, but in doing so, the osseous blood supply can potentially be compromised. In certain talar neck and body fracture scenarios, an arthroscopic approach has been described. Hawkins II talar neck fractures with minimal displacement and 2-part body fractures without severe soft tissue compromise can be reduced and fixated using an arthroscopic-assisted approach.[25,48] For the approach, standard anteromedial and anterolateral ankle portals are used with either a 4.0- or 2.7-mm arthroscope with gravity inflow. This approach allows visualization of the entire neck and body and evaluation for varus rotation of the fracture. In addition, lateral neck comminution can be visualized. Distraction of the ankle manually and plantarflexion of the foot allow the arthroscope to be passed between the fracture fragments and into the subtalar joint for visualization and removal of any chondral debris.[48] Alternatively, lateral subtalar portals can be placed for visualization of the lateral subtalar joint.[29] Direct reduction of the fracture is visualized through the ankle joint, and temporary stabilization is placed. Screw fixation is achieved with 3.5- or 4.0-mm titanium screws in the anterior-posterior direction. The screws ideally should be placed perpendicular to the fracture line. In order to achieve this orientation, screws are typically placed anteriorly from the dorsomedial and anterolateral aspects of the talar neck or starting in the dorsal aspect of the articular surface of the talar head and directed into the body. If screws are started in the articular surface, then they should be adequately countersunk. Saltzman and colleagues[48] described a case of a comminuted talar body fracture in which arthroscopy was used to assist in reduction and internal fixation. No wound complication occurred, and at 6 months postoperatively, the patient had resumed normal activity with mild symptomatic pain. Wajsfisz and colleagues[49] described the use arthroscopy in a Hawkins III talar neck fracture using 4 portals and cannulated screws. No complications were reported.

CALCANEAL FRACTURES

Calcaneal fractures encompass 2% of all fractures, most being intra-articular.[50] They are most commonly treated with ORIF using an extensile lateral or sinus tarsi incisional approach.[51–53] Certain fracture patterns (tongue-type) are amenable to percutaneous reduction and fixation.[54–57] Open approaches, specifically the extensile lateral approach, have well-documented complications, most notably wound healing, dehiscence, and deep infection.[58,59] Regardless of approach, the goals of surgical treatment remain the same. The surgical tactic is to reduce the varus rotation of the tuberosity, to reduce lateral wall blowout, and to restore the calcaneal height and articular congruity. A stepwise approach to these injuries is required in order to achieve reduction and deliver appropriate fixation. An arthroscopically assisted approach can be used for simpler intra-articular fracture patterns with smaller amounts of displacement. This would include mainly Sanders type II fractures (**Fig. 15**).[57,60] The authors recommend a small incision approach for these scenarios over the sinus tarsi. This allows direct visualization of the posterior facet of the subtalar joint. A small joint (2.7-mm or 1.9-mm arthroscope) can be delivered into the wound to assess the articular surface and fracture lines. A transcalcaneal Schanz pin is then inserted into the tuber, and the Essex-Lopresti maneuver performed to correct the heel varus. Provisional smooth wires are then placed from the tuberosity fragment obliquely in the sustentacular fragment. The posterior facet is then reduced so no articular step-offs exist (**Fig. 16**). Reduction should be checked with the image intensifier and visualized with the

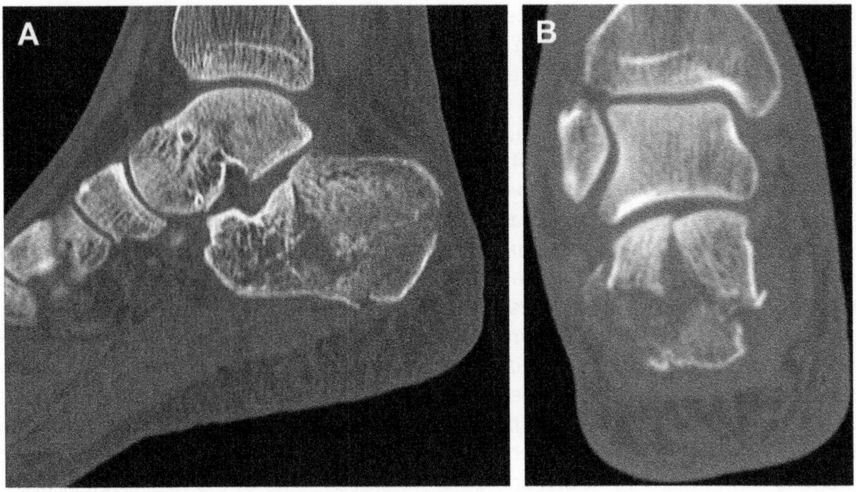

Fig. 15. (*A*) Sagittal CT of Sanders type II calcaneus fracture. (*B*) Frontal CT with articular "step-off" of the posterior subtalar facet.

arthroscope. Often what appears to be anatomic on imaging is slightly malreduced when visualized with the arthroscope.

Gavlik and colleagues[56] published a series of 15 patients examining the posterior facet during hardware removal. Fifteen patients presented for hardware removal after previously undergoing ORIF for intra-articular calcaneal fractures, 7 of which had at least a 1-mm step-off within the posterior facet. In 25% of cases using fluoroscopy to judge reduction during ORIF, arthroscopy detected incongruency in the posterior calcaneal facet. They determined that arthroscopy is a useful tool to detect incongruency, reduces time of intraoperative fluoroscopy, is more precise than fluoroscopy, and permits fragment removal. If the surgeon is pleased with the reduction from a fluoroscopic and arthroscopic standpoint, then definitive fixation can be delivered. The authors prefer delivering thalamic screws first in an oblique orientation to stabilize the posterior facet fragments. Rafting screws can be delivered from the tuberosity fragment to the sustentacular fragment. Last, a lateral plate can be inserted to connect the posterior facet to the anterolateral fragment.

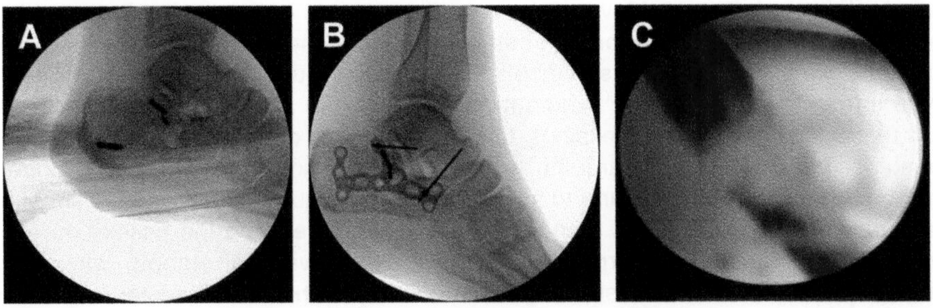

Fig. 16. (*A, B*) Reduction sequence of a joint depression calcaneal fracture. (*C*) Arthroscopic visualization of horizontal fracture line through the posterior facet.

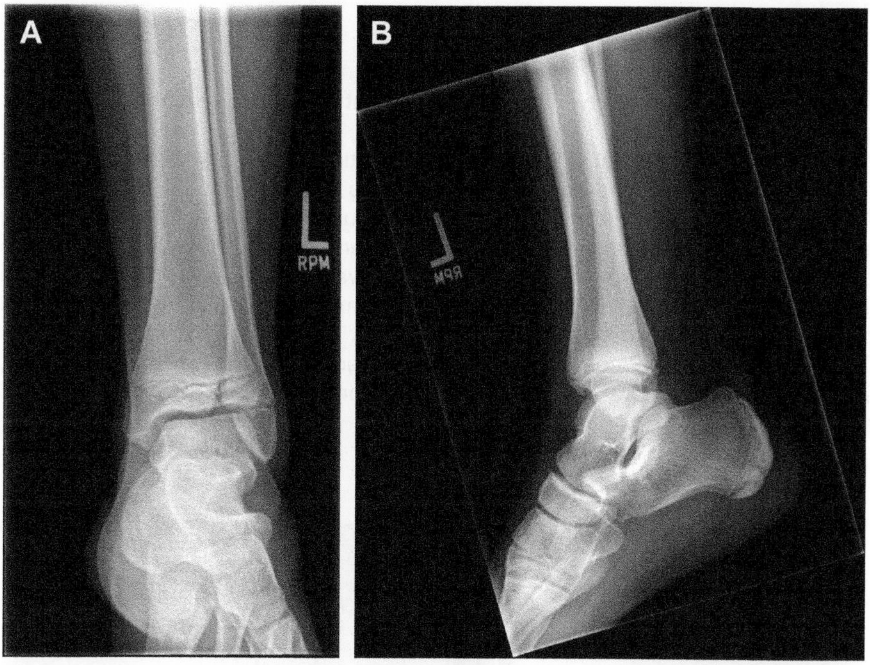

Fig. 17. (*A*) AP radiograph of a Tillaux fracture. (*B*) Preoperative lateral radiograph.

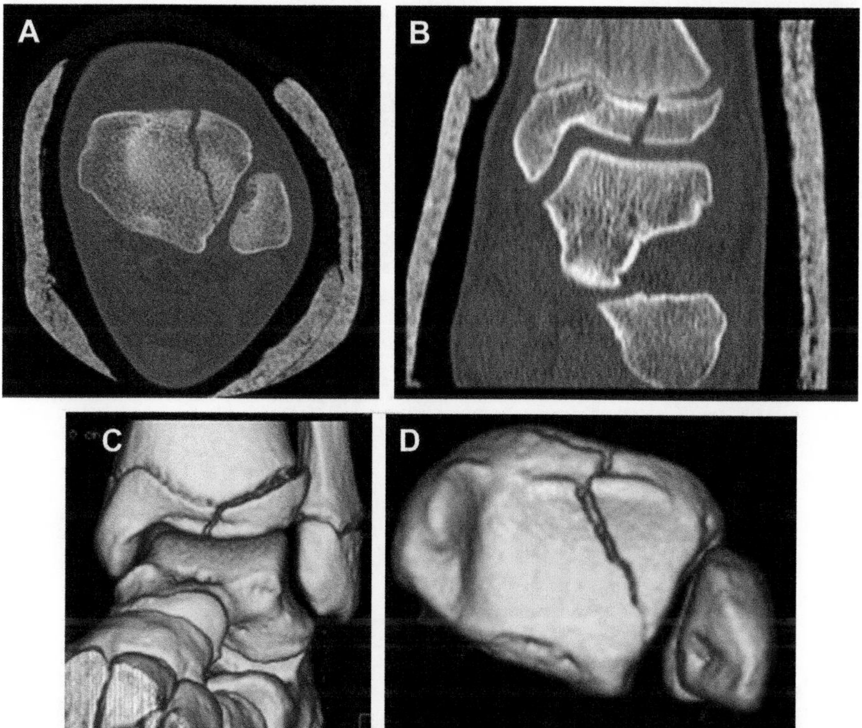

Fig. 18. (*A*) Axial CT with lateral displacement. (*B*) Frontal plane CT scan showing the quadrilateral shape of the fragment and lateral displacement. (*C*) 3D reconstructed CT. (*D*) Inferior view of the fracture showing lateral displacement.

Other investigators have favorable results without a small incision, but using standard sinus tarsi portals.

Rammelt and colleagues[60] looked at 61 patients with Sanders II calcaneal fractures. They were treated with percutaneous reduction and internal fixation. Arthroscopy was used to confirm anatomic reduction of the subtalar joint using a 2.7-mm arthroscope and standard portals. There were no wound complications or infections. Schuberth and colleagues[54] evaluated patients with Sanders II and III injuries intraoperatively using a 4.0-mm 70° arthroscope using a lateral portal over the sinus tarsi. A second portal was used directly over the posterior facet. All cases used fluoroscopy to visualize reduction, and in 10 of 24 cases, an arthroscope was used. No wound complications, infections, or nerve irritations occurred.

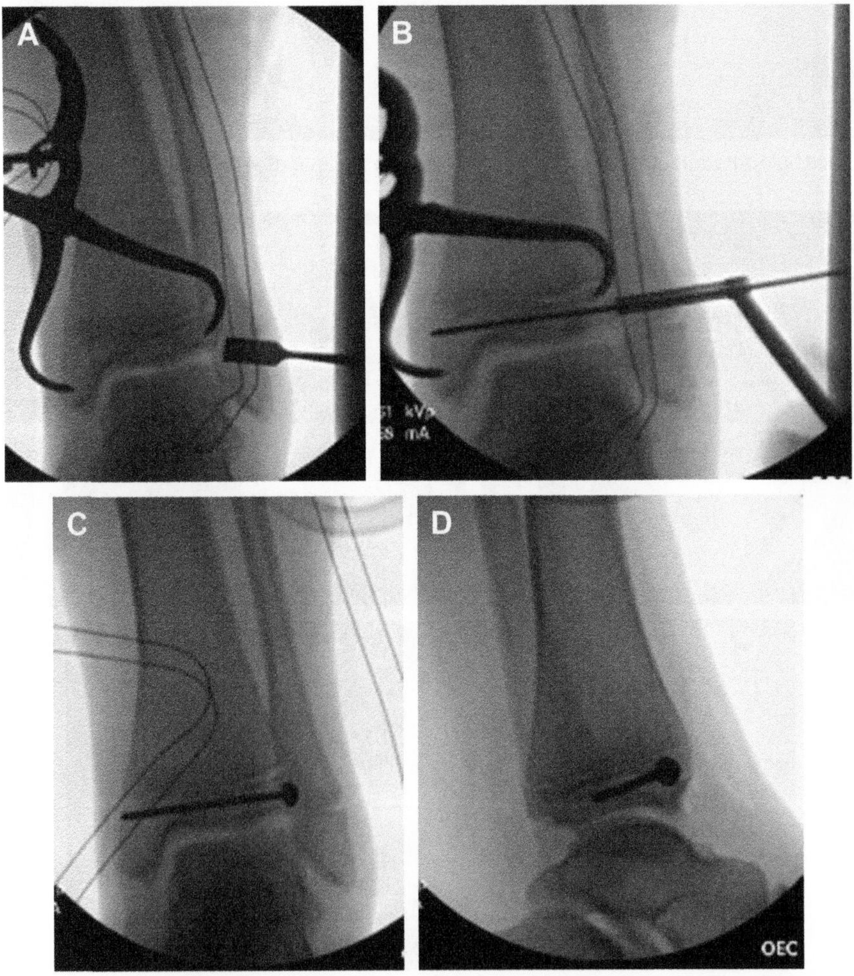

Fig. 19. (*A*) Percutaneous reduction of the laterally displaced fracture fragment. (*B*) Temporary stabilization with a K-wire after reduction. (*C*) AP view showing definitive fixation. (*D*) Lateral view with definitive fixation using a single lag screw with a washer.

PEDIATRIC ANKLE FRACTURES

Almost 40% of physeal injuries occur in the ankle.[61] Tibial fractures are the second most common physeal fracture. Asymmetric closure of the distal tibia finishes at age 15 in girls and 17 in boys. Closure occurs over an 18-month period, which begins centrally and progresses medially, with the anterolateral aspect closing last. This asymmetric closure commonly leads to transitional fractures, which include juvenile Tillaux and triplane fractures. Surgical treatment is indicated in intra-articular fractures in which displacement is greater than 2 mm.[62,63]

JUVENILE TILLAUX FRACTURE

A Tillaux injury almost always occurs in the adolescent within a year of complete closure of the distal tibial physis. The injury is a Salter-Harris III fracture in which the lateral portion of the distal tibial physis is injured.[63,64] The central and medial aspects of the tibial physis have closed, leaving the anterolateral aspect open and vulnerable to injury. An external rotation force on the foot may avulse the anterolateral quadrant of the tibial physis, which is bound to the fibula by the strong anterior tibiofibular ligament, resulting in a rectangular or pie-shaped fragment being broken off the distal tibial physis. This pie-shaped fragment is displaced and rotated laterally with a gap separating the fragment but normally without articular step-off (**Fig. 17**). A CT scan best demonstrates this fracture (**Fig. 18**). An arthroscopic approach can easily visualize the fracture along the anterior aspect of the tibia and allow for debridement of the hematoma. A percutaneously placed large pointed reduction forceps can reduce the fracture

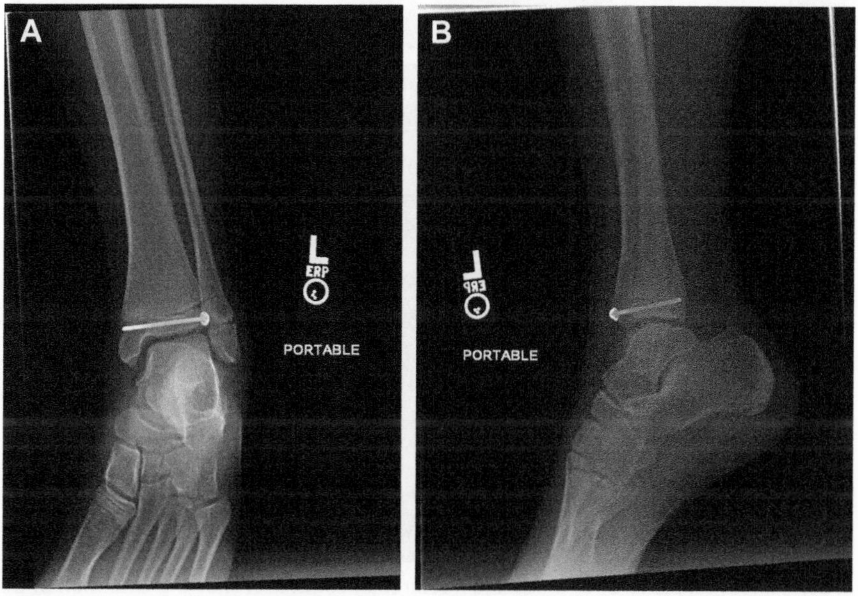

Fig. 20. (*A*) Postoperative AP radiograph with stable fixation and reduction of the fracture. (*B*) Postoperative lateral radiograph.

under arthroscopic and fluoroscopic visualization. A cannulated lag screw can then be delivered percutaneously under fluoroscopic control (**Fig. 19**). The screw can be perpendicular to the ankle joint or angled slightly superiorly. Crossing the epiphyseal plate with a screw is not an issue because this is the last portion to close (**Fig. 20**). Leetun and Ireland[65] first reported arthroscopic-assisted reduction of a Tillaux fracture in a 14 year old. The fracture and articular surface were directly visualized. Arthroscopy was used to confirm reduction. Jennings and colleagues[66] treated a single patient in their case series of juvenile epiphyseal fractures with a fully threaded cortical lag screw. Five years after the injury, radiographs were negative for arthritis, and motion was unrestricted.

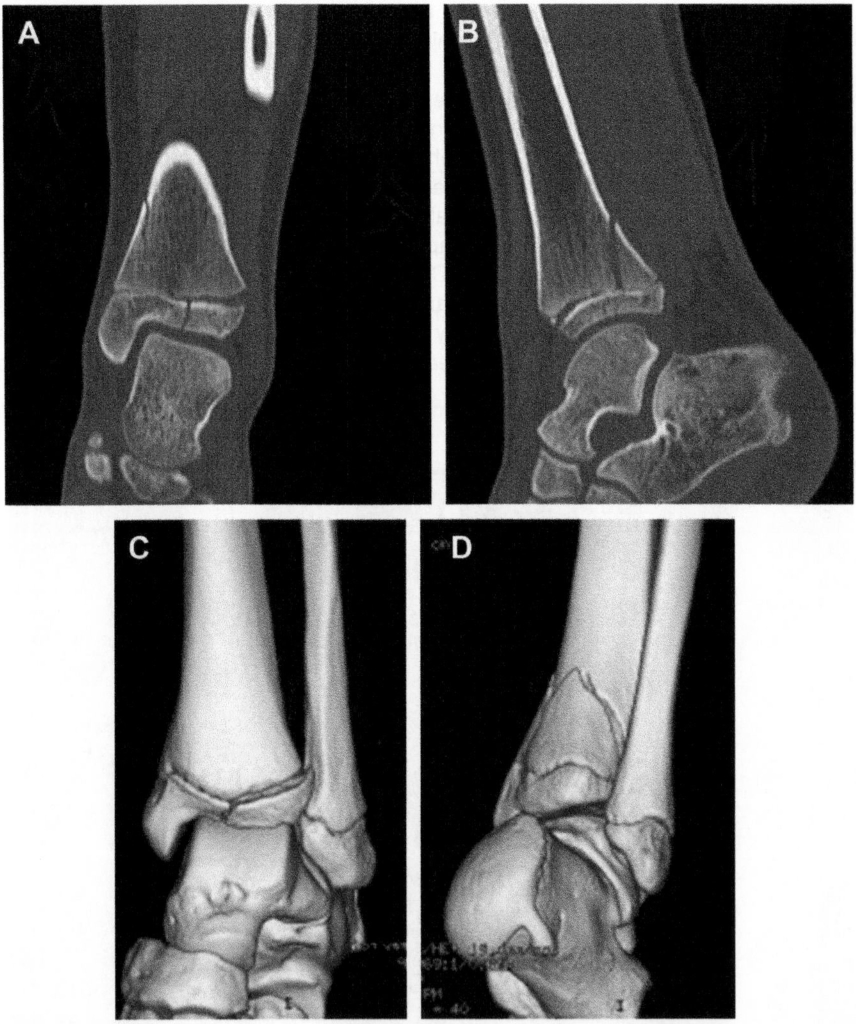

Fig. 21. (*A*) Frontal plane CT of a triplane fracture. (*B*) Sagittal CT showing extension of the fracture into the metaphysis. (*C*) 3D reconstructed CT of a triplane fracture. (*D*) 3D reconstruction showing posterior metaphyseal spike.

TRIPLANE FRACTURE

The tibial triplane fracture is a complex fracture defined by sagittal, transverse, and coronal components that course in part along, and in part through, the physis, finally entering the ankle joint. The mechanism of injury is external rotation along with pronation and plantarflexion.[63,64,67] It is seen in children slightly younger than for the Tillaux fracture. It is classically described as a combination Salter-Harris type II in the metaphysis and type III fracture in the epiphysis. It extends from the ankle joint across the epiphysis through the epiphyseal plate, progressing into the metaphysis. Perhaps it should best be thought of as a variation type IV fracture. This fracture requires a CT scan for evaluation to assess fracture displacement and articular "step-off" (**Fig. 21**). Fracture patterns vary, and usually one can identify 2 or 3 parts, although 4 parts have been reported. Operative treatment is recommended if the displacement is 2 mm or more, and for articular "step-off" or incongruity. The degree of displacement can vary greatly in these injuries. If the displacement is not too large, then the triplane fracture can be approached as described for the Tillaux fracture with arthroscopically assisted percutaneous reduction and internal fixation (**Fig. 22**). Arthroscopic visualization of the fracture line anteriorly along the tibia is usually good. One or 2 lag screws are placed in the epiphysis depending on the number of fragments, followed by 1 or 2 screws in the metaphyseal component (**Fig. 23**). If the displacement is large, then a closed reduction will be necessary to bring the fracture fragments into closer apposition. Then, an arthroscopically assisted percutaneous method can be used. In certain cases, incarcerated periosteum can thwart this approach and will then require ORIF. In 1993, Whipple and colleagues[68] reported 2 patients with 2-part triplane fractures. Both patients went on to union with no complications. They concluded that arthroscopy reduces surgical trauma, allows fracture visualization, and ensures reduction and congruity under direct visualization. Imade and colleagues[69] described arthroscopic-assisted reduction with percutaneous fixation in a 14-year-old boy who sustained a triplane injury with more than 5 mm of displacement. The arthroscope was used to assess the fracture site. One year postoperatively, an arthroscope was then used to assess the ankle joint articular surface, which was noted to be congruous. In the largest case series, Jennings and colleagues[66] treated 5 triplane fractures with arthroscopic assistance and a minimum follow-up of 1 year.

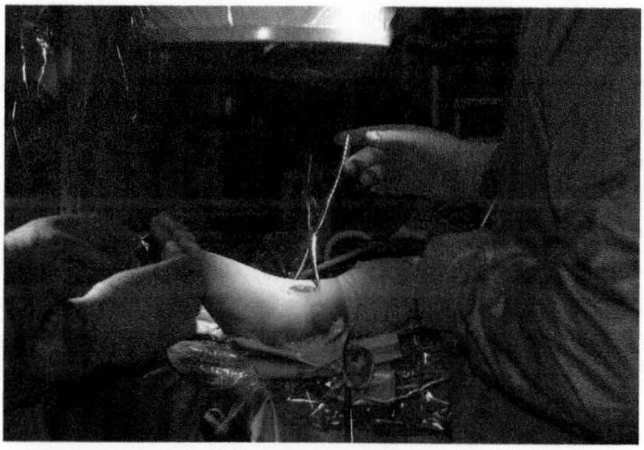

Fig. 22. Intraoperative, percutaneously clamp reduction.

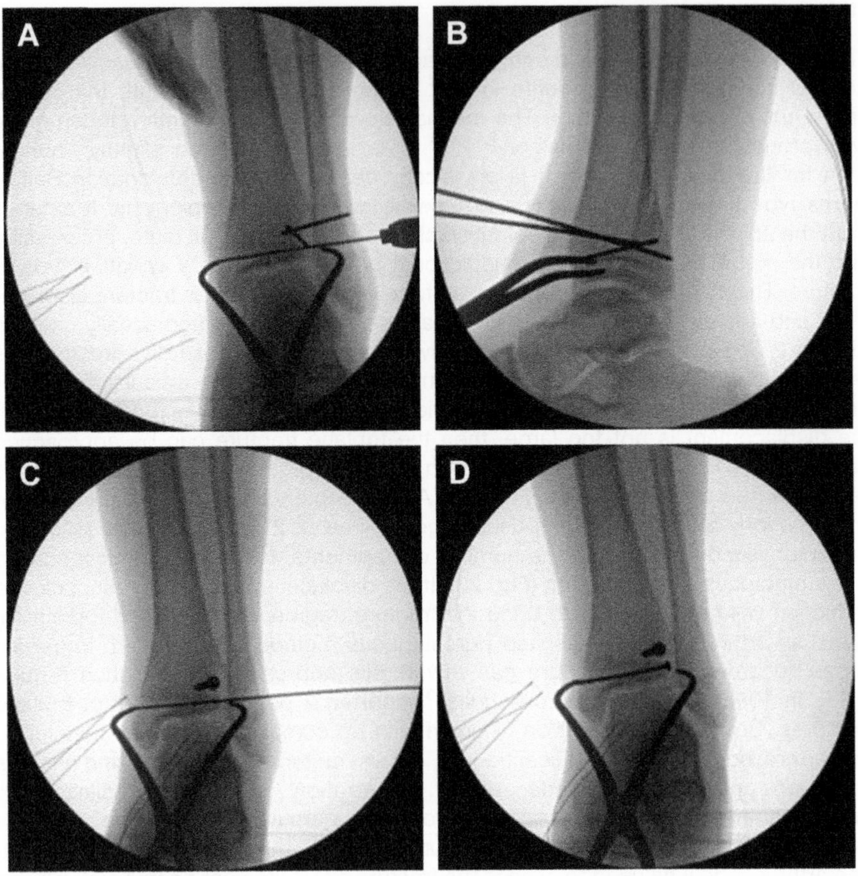

Fig. 23. (*A*) Percutaneous reduction and temporary stabilization. (*B*) Temporary stabilization of the metaphyseal fracture fragment. (*C*) Introduction of K-wire into the distal aspect of the fracture for stabilization. (*D*) Fluoroscopic imaging showing percutaneous reduction and screw fixation.

SUMMARY

Arthroscopy is an immensely valuable surgical tool in assisting with fracture reduction and fixation. Access to the joint can be gained either through the surgical wound or through standard portals. These minimal incisions preserve the periosteal blood supply and potentially afford a fast recovery time for the patient. Gravity inflow is recommended and provides adequate distention and visualization without excessive fluid extravasation into the soft tissues. Initial debridement of the joint debris and hematoma is almost always required. This can be accomplished with a high-speed shaver. The surgeon can now inspect the entire joint and remove fracture debris that ordinarily would have been left alone. Articular injury can be documented and potentially treated. With the aid of reduction clamps and/or K-wires, under direct visualization, the surgeon can achieve near precise anatomic reduction of the articular surface.

REFERENCES

1. Jackson RW. A history of arthroscopy. Arthroscopy 2010;26:91–103.

2. Takagi K. The classic. Arthroscope. Kenji Takagi. J. Jap. Orthop. Assoc., 1939. Clin Orthop Relat Res 1982;(167):6–8.
3. Burman MS. Arthroscopy of direct visualization of joints. An experimental cadaver study. J Bone Joint Surg 1931;13:669–95.
4. Watanabe M. Arthroscopy of small joints. Tokyo: Igaku-Shoin; 1982.
5. Drez D, Guhl JF, Gollehan DL. Ankle arthroscopy: technique and indications. Clin Sports Med 1982;1:35–45.
6. Heller AS, Vogler HW. Ankle joint arthroscopy. J Foot Surg 1982;21:23–9.
7. Lundeen RO. Arthroscopic anatomy of the anterior aspect of the ankle. J Am Podiatr Med Assoc 1985;75:372–6.
8. Parisien JS, Vangsness T. Arthroscopy of the subtalar joint: an experimental approach. Arthroscopy 1985;1(1):53–7.
9. Atesok K, Doral MN, Whipple T, et al. Arthroscopy-assisted fracture fixation. Knee Surg Sports Traumatol Arthrosc 2011;19(2):320–9.
10. Ferkel RD, Scranton PE. Current concepts review: arthroscopy of the ankle and foot. J Bone Joint Surg Am 1993;75(8):1233–42.
11. Glazebrook MA, Ganapathy V, Bridge MA, et al. Evidence-based indications for ankle arthroscopy. Arthroscopy 2009;25(12):1478–90.
12. Marcus RE, Balourdas GM, Heiple KG. Ankle arthrodesis by chevron fusion with internal fixation and bone grafting. J Bone Joint Surg Am 2007;89:1899–905.
13. Loren GJ, Ferkel RD. Arthroscopic assessment of occult intra-articular injury in acute ankle fractures. Arthroscopy 1997;18:412–21.
14. Hintermann B, Regazzoni P, Lampert C, et al. Arthroscopic findings in acute fracture of the ankle. J Bone Joint Surg Br 2000;82:345–51.
15. Thordarson DB, Bains R, Shepher LE. The role of ankle arthroscopy on the surgical management of ankle fractures. Foot Ankle Int 2001;22(2):123–5.
16. Ono A, Nishikawa S, Nagao A, et al. Arthroscopically assisted treatment of ankle fractures: arthroscopic findings and surgical outcomes. Arthroscopy 2004;20: 627–31.
17. Leontaritis N, Hinojosa L, Panchbhavi VK. Arthroscopically detected intra-articular lesions associated with acute ankle fractures. J Bone Joint Surg Am 2009;91(2):33–9.
18. Pires RE, Mauffrey C, De Andrade MA, et al. Minimally invasive percutaneous plate osteosynthesis for ankle fractures: a prospective observational cohort study. Eur J Orthop Surg Traumatol 2014;24(7):1297–303.
19. Takao M, Ochi M, Shu N, et al. Bandage distraction technique for ankle arthroscopy. Foot Ankle Int 1999;20:389.
20. Michelson JD. Current concepts review: fractures of the ankle. J Bone Joint Surg Am 1990;77:142–52.
21. Beris AE, Kabbani KT, Xenakis TA, et al. Surgical treatment of malleolar fractures. A review of 144 patients. Clin Orthop Relat Res 1997;341:91–8.
22. Davidovitch RI, Walsh M, Spitzer A, et al. Functional outcome after operatively treated ankle fractures in the elderly. Foot Ankle Int 2009;30(8):728–33.
23. Egol KA, Tejwani NC, Walsh MG, et al. Predictors of short-term functional outcome following ankle fracture surgery. J Bone Joint Surg Am 2006;88(5): 974–9.
24. Lindsjo U. Operative treatment of ankle fracture-dislocations: a follow-up study of 306/321 consecutive cases. Clin Orthop Relat Res 1985;199:28–38.
25. Bonasia DE, Rossi R, Saltzman CL, et al. The role of arthroscopy in the management of fractures about the ankle. J Am Acad Orthop Surg 2011;19:226–35.

26. Dawe EJ, Jukes CP, Ganesan K, et al. Ankle arthroscopy to manage sequelae after ankle fractures. Knee Surg Sports Traumatol Arthrosc 2015;23(11):3393–7.
27. Utsugi K, Sakai H, Hiraoka H, et al. Intra-articular fibrous tissue formation following ankle fracture: the significance of arthroscopic debridement of fibrous tissue. Arthroscopy 2007;23(1):89–93.
28. Pankovich AM. Maisonneuve fracture of the fibula. J Bone Joint Surg Am 1976;58: 337.
29. Wood DA, Christensen JC, Schuberth JM. The use of arthroscopy in acute foot and ankle trauma. Foot Ankle Spec 2014;7(6):495–506.
30. Ferkel RD, Orwin JF. Ankle arthroscopy: a new tool for treating acute and chronic ankle fractures. Arthroscopy 1993;9:456.
31. Ruedi T, Allgower M. Fractures of the lower end of the tibia into the ankle joint. Clin Orthop 1979;138:105–10.
32. Mast JW, Spiegel PG, Pappas JN. Fractures of the tibial pilon. Clin Orthop 1988; 230:68–82.
33. Tornetta P, Weiner L, Bergman M, et al. Pilon fractures: treatment with combined internal and external fixation. J Orthop Trauma 1993;7:489–96.
34. Sirkin M, Sanders R, DiPasquale T, et al. A staged protocol for soft tissue management in the treatment of complex pilon fractures. J Orthop Trauma 1999;13: 78–84.
35. Chen SH, Wu PH, Lee YS. Long-term results of pilon fractures. Arch Orthop Trauma Surg 2007;127:55–60.
36. Jansen H, Fenwick A, Doht S, et al. Clinical outcome and changes in gait pattern after pilon fractures. Int Orthop 2013;37(1):51–8.
37. Korkmaz A, Ciftdemir M, Ozcan M, et al. The analysis of the variables, affecting outcome in surgically treated tibia pilon fractured patients. Injury 2013;44(10): 1270–4.
38. Hammond AW, Crist BD. Arthroscopic management of C3 tibial plafond fractures: a technical guide. J Foot Ankle Surg 2012;51:382–6.
39. Leonard M, Magill P, Khayyat G. Minimally-invasive treatment of high velocity intra-articular fractures of the distal tibia. Int Orthop 2009;33(4):1149–53.
40. Salton HL, Rush S, Schuberth J. Tibial plafond fractures: limited incision reduction with percutaneous fixation. J Foot Ankle Surg 2007;46(4):261–9.
41. Kralinger F, Lutz M, Wambacher M, et al. Arthroscopically assisted reconstruction and percutaneous screw fixation of a Pilon tibial fracture. Arthroscopy 2003;19(5): 1–4.
42. Mulfinger GL, Trueta J. The blood supply to the talus. J Bone Joint Surg Br 1970; 52:160–7.
43. Hawkins LG. Fractures of the neck of the talus. J Bone Joint Surg Am 1970;52: 991–1002.
44. Canale ST, Kelly FB. Fractures of the neck of the talus. J Bone Joint Surg Am 1978;60:143–56.
45. Vallier HA, Nork SE, Barei DP, et al. Talar neck fractures: results and outcomes. J Bone Joint Surg Am 2004;86(8):1616–24.
46. Mayo KA. Fractures of the talus: principles of management and techniques of treatment. Tech Orthop 1987;2:42–54.
47. Berlet GC, Lee TH, Massa EG. Talar neck fractures. Orthop Clin North Am 2001; 32:53–64.
48. Saltzman CL, Marsh JL, Tearse DS. Treatment of displaced talus fractures: an arthroscopically assisted approach. Foot Ankle Int 1994;15(11):630–3.

49. Wajsfisz A, Makridis KG, Guillou R, et al. Arthroscopic treatment of a talar neck fracture: a case report. Knee Surg Sports Traumatol Arthrosc 2012;20:1850–3.
50. Csizy M, Buckley R, Tough S, et al. Displaced intra-articular calcaneal fractures: variables predicting late subtalar fusion. J Orthop Trauma 2003;17:106–12.
51. Zwipp H, Tscherne H, Thermann H, et al. Osteosynthesis of displaced intraarticular fractures of the calcaneus. Results in 123 cases. Clin Orthop 1993;290: 76–86.
52. Benirschke SK, Sangeorzan BJ. Extensive intra-articular fractures of the foot. Surgical management of calcaneal fractures. Clin Orthop Relat Res 1993;292: 128–34.
53. Sanders R, Fortin P, DiPasquale T, et al. Operative treatment in 120 displaced intraarticular calcaneal fractures. Results using a prognostic computed tomography scan classification. Clin Orthop Relat Res 2002;290:87–95.
54. Schuberth JM, Cobb MD, Talarico RH. Minimally invasive arthroscopic-assisted reduction with percutaneous fixation in the management of intra-articular calcaneal fractures: a review of 24 cases. J Foot Ankle Surg 2009;48(3):315–22.
55. Nehme A, Chaminade B, Chiron P, et al. Percutaneous fluoroscopic and arthroscopic controlled screw fixation of posterior facet fractures of the calcaneus. Rev Chir Orthop Reparatrice Appar Mot 1998;90:256–64.
56. Gavlik JM, Rammelt S, Zwipp H. Percutaneous, arthroscopically-assisted osteosynthesis of calcaneus fractures. Arch Orthop Trauma Surg 2002;122:424–8.
57. Rammelt S, Amlang M, Barthel S, et al. Minimally-invasive treatment of calcaneal fractures. Injury 2004;35(Suppl 2):55–63.
58. Harvey EJ, Grujic L, Early JS, et al. Morbidity associated with ORIF of intra-articular calcaneus fractures using a lateral approach. Foot Ankle Int 2001;22: 868–73.
59. Abidi NA, Dhawan S, Gruen GS, et al. Wound-healing risk factors after open reduction and internal fixation of calcaneal fractures. Foot Ankle Int 1998;19: 856–61.
60. Rammelt S, Amlang M, Barthel S, et al. Percutaneous treatment of less severe intraarticular calcaneal fractures. Clin Orthop Relat Res 2010;468:983–90.
61. Goldberg VM, Aadalen R. Distal tibial epiphyseal injuries: the role of athletics in fifty-three cases. Am J Sports Med 1978;6:263–8.
62. Herman MJ, MacEwen GD. Physeal fractures of the distal tibia on fibula. Curr Othrop 2003;17:56–62.
63. Spiegel PG, Cooperman DR, Laros GS. Epiphyseal fractures of the distal ends of the tibia and fibula. A retrospective study of two hundred and thirty-seven cases in children. J Bone Joint Surg Am 1978;60A:1046–50.
64. Kleiger B, Mankin HJ. Fracture of the lateral portion of the distal tibia epiphysis. J Bone Joint Surg Am 1964;46:25–32.
65. Leetun DT, Ireland ML. Arthroscopically assisted reduction and fixation of a juvenile Tillaux fracture. Arthroscopy 2002;18(4):427–9.
66. Jennings MM, Lagaay P, Schuberth JM. Arthroscopic assisted fixation of juvenile intra-articular epiphyseal ankle fractures. J Foot Ankle Surg 2007;46(5):376–86.
67. von Laer L. Classification, diagnosis and treatment of transitional fractures of the distal part of the tibia. J Bone Joint Surg Am 1985;67A:687–98.
68. Whipple TL, Martin DR, McIntyre LF, et al. Arthroscopic treatment of triplane fractures of the ankle. Arthroscopy 1993;9(4):456–63.
69. Imade S, Takao M, Nishi H, et al. Arthroscopy-assisted reduction and percutaneous fixation for triplane fracture of the distal tibia. Arthroscopy 2004;20:123–8.

[illegible]

Minimally Invasive Plate Osteosynthesis for Distal Tibia Fractures

Ted C. Lai, DPM[a,*], Justin J. Fleming, DPM[b]

KEYWORDS

• Minimally invasive • MIPO • Distal tibia fracture • Pilon fracture • Percutaneous

KEY POINTS

- Surgical treatment of distal tibia fractures can be a significant challenge associated with many complications.
- Minimally invasive plate osteosynthesis has provided an alternative fixation method with significantly less wound complications than standard open reduction internal fixation.
- Initial evaluation and work up are significantly important because this is a key step with surgical planning. In this phase, it is important to rule out emergent situations, obtain proper reduction along with staging the procedure, and appropriately respect the soft tissue before definitive surgery.
- Minimally invasive plate osteosynthesis displays favorable outcomes in regard to soft tissue and osseous healing, function, and decreased complications.

INTRODUCTION

Distal tibia fractures are devastating injuries that are usually due to high-energy mechanisms such as falling from heights or motor vehicle accidents. They may also occur from low-energy mechanisms, which are seen in rotational injuries around the ankle.[1] Distal tibia and pilon fractures are inherently difficult injuries of the lower extremity to treat owing to the complexity of the fracture along with the sparse soft tissue envelope. In conjunction with significant osseous injury, the surrounding soft tissue structures often become severely traumatized. Owing to the limited subcutaneous layer surrounding the injury, surgical treatment is often prone to developing complications such as wounds, infections, malunion, and nonunion.[1] Historically, wound complications have been documented to be as high as 36% after open reduction internal fixation (ORIF) of distal tibia and pilon fractures, with infections reported as high as 37% to 55%.[2,3]

Disclosure Statement: The authors have nothing to disclose.
[a] Foot and Ankle Surgery, Shore Orthopaedic University Associates, 24 MacArthur Boulevard, Somers Point, NJ 08244, USA; [b] University Orthopaedic Associates, 2 World's Fair Drive, Somerset, NJ 08873, USA
* Corresponding author. 205 Cambridge Avenue, Linwood, NJ 08221.
E-mail address: Ted.C.Lai@gmail.com

Clin Podiatr Med Surg 35 (2018) 223–232
https://doi.org/10.1016/j.cpm.2017.12.005
podiatric.theclinics.com

Distal tibia fracture has been treated in various manners, including intramedullary nailing (IMN), external fixation, ORIF, and minimally invasive plate osteosynthesis (MIPO). One of the more readily used methods for fixation of distal tibia fractures is antegrade IMN. Studies have shown it to be a reliable fixation method but it does present with some significant complications.[4] IMN for distal tibia fractures has displayed morbidity to the knee, which has been reported as high as 71%. Chronic anterior knee pain is among the most common issues, reported to be as high as 73.2%.[5] IMN for distal tibia fractures has also shown to have a significantly increased rate of malalignment compared with plate fixation.[4]

ORIF is another frequently used method of treatment of distal tibia fractures. ORIF can be performed with many different incisional approaches. The anterolateral approach is more frequently used. The anterolateral incision is performed at the anterior ankle, which is an area historically known to have poor healing. The extensive dissection required for visualization and reduction of the fracture disrupts the surrounding soft tissue and extraosseous vascular supply. Often, the dissection devitalizes the fracture fragments.[6] This has been known to delay healing and, ultimately, may contribute to the development of nonunion. The extensive dissection involved with ORIF, especially with the anterolateral approach, has displayed increased results of wound complications, including dehiscence; full-thickness necrosis; and, ultimately, infection (**Fig. 1**). These complications are of significant gravity because

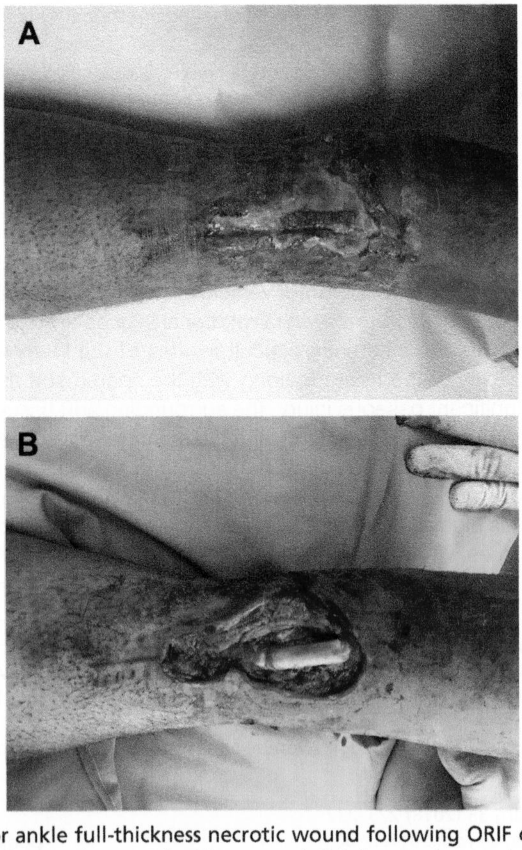

Fig. 1. (*A*) Anterior ankle full-thickness necrotic wound following ORIF of a pilon fracture. (*B*) Debridement of necrotic wound with exposed tibialis anterior tendon and hardware.

they may require use of long-term intravenous antibiotics, multiple visits to the operating room for debridement, and may lead to eventual limb loss.

Percutaneous or MIPO technique for distal tibia fractures is an alternative fixation method. It has decreased the risk of soft tissue complications that were observed in the extensive anterolateral plate osteosynthesis. There have been studies that have demonstrated decreased vascular insult with medial percutaneous plating compared with the standard anterolateral open approach.[7] MIPO also presents without the risk of complications to the knee, as well as less chance of developing malalignment of the fracture compared with IMN. MIPO provides appropriate anatomic reduction and stability to the fracture, maintains a biologically friendly environment for fracture healing, and decreases wound complications through the creation of smaller incisions. Many studies have reported similar outcomes with fewer complications of MIPO compared with IMN and open approach.[6,8]

INDICATIONS

MIPO for distal tibia fractures is better suited for patients who have a less than optimal soft tissue envelope where extensive dissection would carry high risk for wound complications. The MIPO technique is more reserved for fractures to the distal tibia in which the plafond does not present with severe comminution. In cases in which significant disruption and comminution of the tibial plafond is involved, MIPO may not be able to adequately restore the articular surface. These fractures would be better served with either ORIF through the anterolateral approach; alternative incisional approaches that give direct exposure to the articular surface; or, ultimately, primary fusion.

Fracture pattern and deformity also plays a role in selection of plating technique. Distal tibia fractures with varus deformity are better treated with medial buttress plating. Medial buttress plating will better counter the deforming forces and provide an overall stronger construct (**Fig. 2**).

CONTRAINDICATIONS

Situations that would not be optimal with use of MIPO include soft tissue defects or compromise of the medial ankle or distal leg, fractures in which severe comminution of the distal tibia and plafond are involved, or vascular compromise or injury to the surrounding area.

EVALUATION AND WORKUP

The patient is initially evaluated in the emergency department and treated according to the trauma protocol. The lower extremity is evaluated to confirm patent neurovascular status and to rule out compartment syndrome. Open fractures are treated appropriately with intravenous antibiotics and emergently irrigated and debrided. Depending on the severity and instability of the fracture, closed reduction is performed and maintained with either a well-padded splint or with application of a spanning external fixator.

Spanning external fixation is performed to reduce the fracture and maintain anatomic alignment to prevent damage to the surrounding soft tissue. It also provides structural stability in the interim to allow for the soft tissue envelope to stabilize. External fixation application in the form of a delta frame is performed by placing 2 5 mm half pins in the anterior aspect of the proximal tibia, making sure pin placement is sufficiently away from the zone of injury and the area of the definitive operative site. A 6 mm transcalcaneal pin is placed through the calcaneal tuber from medial to lateral.

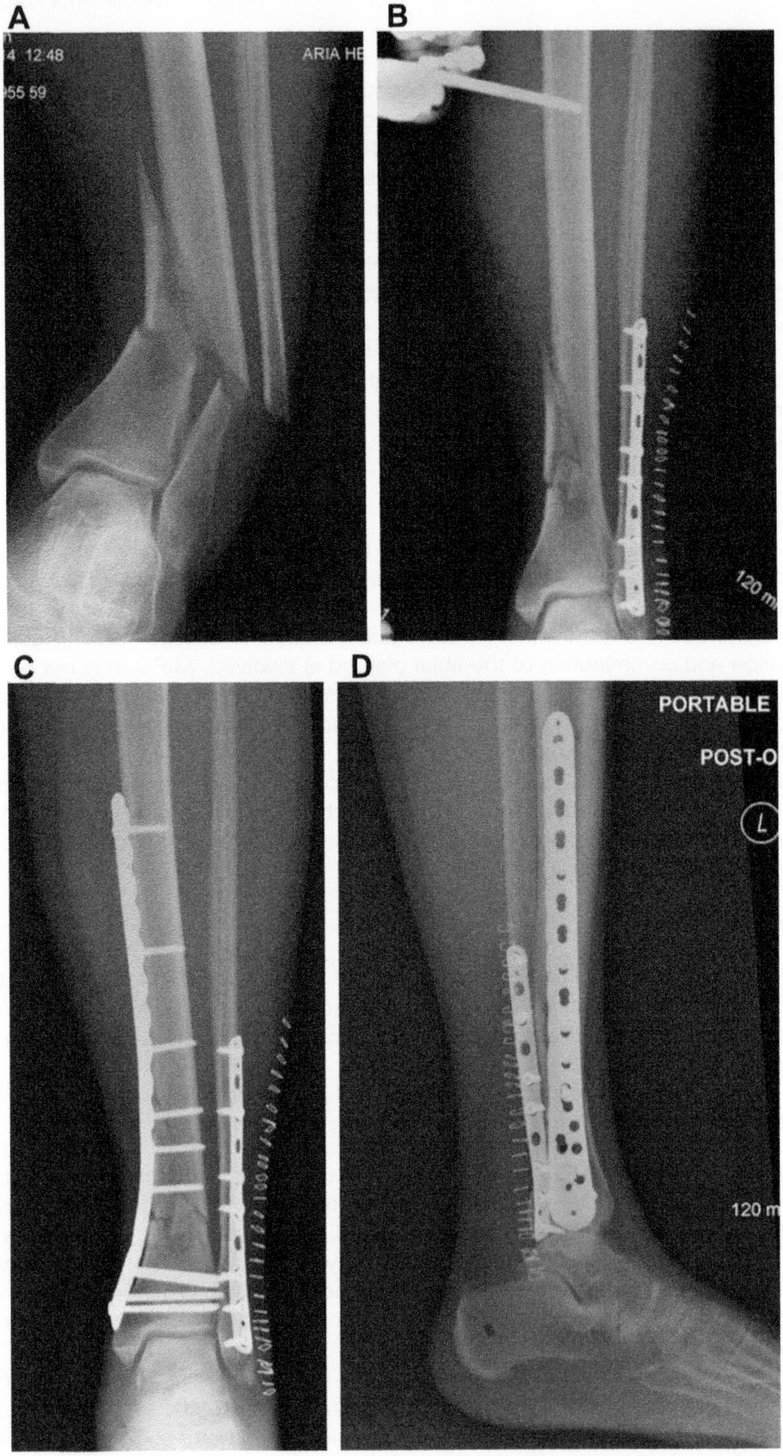

Fig. 2. (*A*) Distal tibia fracture with varus deformity. (*B*) Postreduction of distal tibia fracture with use of delta external fixator along with fibular ORIF. (*C*) Anteroposterior (AP) radiograph of MIPO technique for distal tibia fracture. (*D*) Lateral radiograph of MIPO technique for distal tibia fracture.

Carbon fiber rods are then attached to the pins and traction is applied to bring the tibia out to length, as well as to correct for varus or valgus deformity.

Staging of distal tibia fractures is preferred when possible. In the initial stage, application of the external fixator is performed along with ORIF of the distal fibula fracture if the fracture is present. Fixation of the fibula restores the proper length and provides lateral stability. This allows for adequate time for healing of the soft tissue before definitive fixation of the distal tibia. It also prevents compromise to the soft tissue envelope by not having to make multiple incisions at the time of the definitive surgery (see **Fig. 2**B).

Computed tomography (CT) scan is then performed postreduction for further evaluation, as well as surgical planning of the distal tibia fracture. CT scans should be performed with 1.25 mm slices reoriented to the ankle joint. CT 3-dimensional reconstructions of the tibia can also be obtained to better appreciate the fracture pattern and spatial relationship. Definitive surgery is then delayed until the soft tissue envelope becomes stable, which may range from 7 to 14 days. The soft tissue is noted to be stable for definitive surgery when there is absence of fracture blisters and a positive wrinkle test is present indicating decreased soft tissue swelling.

SURGICAL TECHNIQUE

At the time of definitive surgery, the patient is placed on the operating table in a supine position. The lower extremity, along with the external fixator, is appropriately prepped before draping. Typically, the external fixator is left in place during the procedure to maintain reduction and to aid with manipulation of the distal tibia fracture. Rods from the external fixator may be removed as needed if better exposure is required.

The fracture is reduced with a combination of bone clamps and bone forceps, along with Kirschner wires, then confirmed under fluoroscopic guidance. Once adequate reduction is achieved, an approximately 4 cm vertical incision is made over the medial malleolus. In patients with a thinner soft tissue envelope, a horizontal incision can be made below the level of the medial malleolus. The incision is deepened down through subcutaneous tissue, with care being taken to avoid all major neurovascular structures of the leg. The greater saphenous vein and saphenous nerve will be encountered here. Through this incision, a soft tissue elevator is advanced up the medial aspect of the tibia proximally to create a subcutaneous tunnel, allowing for percutaneous placement of the medial distal tibial plate. Plates can either be bent to better contour the medial aspect of the tibia or an anatomically precontoured medial distal tibia plate can be used. An appropriate sized medial distal tibia plate is then passed through the previously created subcutaneous tunnel in a percutaneous manner. Pliers may be used to gain better leverage to advance the plate proximally along the medial aspect of the tibia. The placement of the plate is identified under fluoroscopy and, once proper placement is achieved, the plate is then temporarily fixated with olive wires or pins through small percutaneous incisions. Plate compressive devices may be used to perform plate-assisted reduction of the tibial fracture. With the use of fluoroscopy, the proximal holes of the plate are identified and multiple small stab incisions are made along the medial aspect of the plate. The stab incisions are dissected bluntly with a hemostat down to the level of the plate and the appropriate holes are identified. Screw fixation is placed across the plate into the lateral cortex of the tibia for bicortical fixation. At least 3 bicortical screws are placed proximal to the fracture and distal to the main portion of the fracture. Additional interfragmentary screws are placed based on the fracture pattern observed on the CT scan (**Fig. 3**).

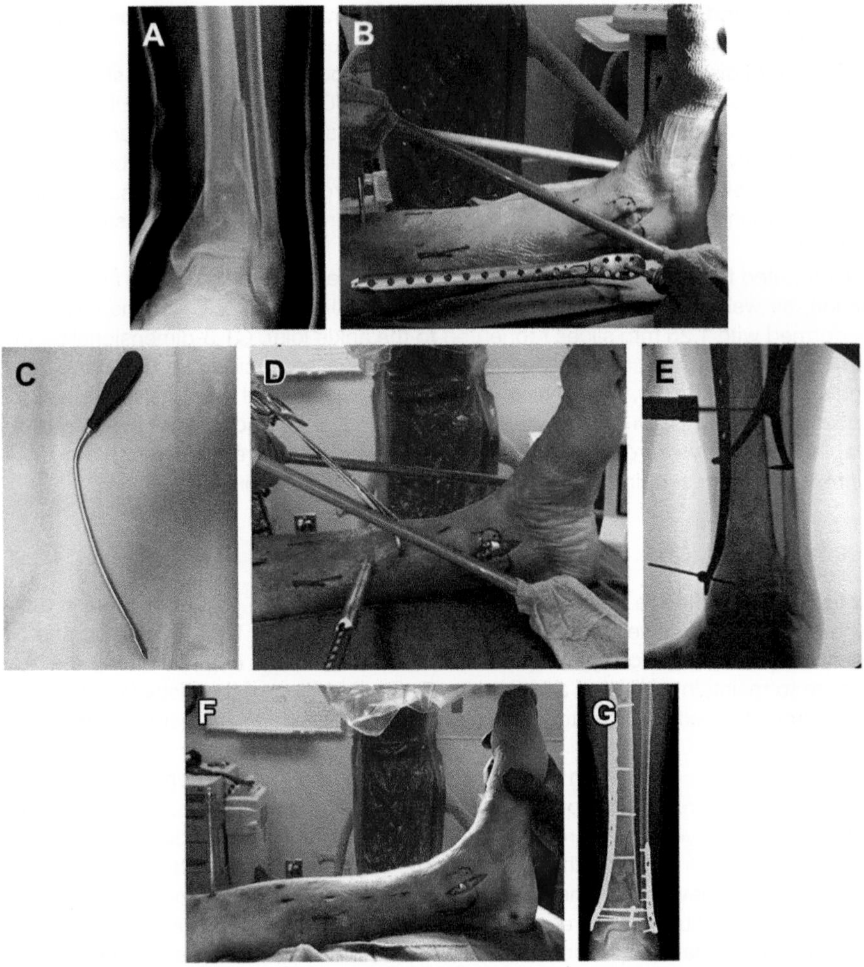

Fig. 3. (*A*) AP radiograph of distal tibia fracture with varus deformity. (*B*) Minimally invasive incision at the medial malleolus with alignment of the medial distal tibia plate on the surface. (*C*) Soft tissue elevator is used to create a subcutaneous tunnel along the medial tibia for percutaneous placement of the plate. (*D*) Medial distal tibia plate is temporarily fixated to the tibia. Percutaneous incisions are made for placement of proximal screws. (*E*) AP fluoroscopy used to aid in percutaneous placement of proximal screws. (*F*) Medial aspect of leg displaying MIPO of a distal tibia fracture. (*G*) AP radiograph of MIPO technique for a distal tibia fracture.

The external fixator is removed and incision sites are then copiously irrigated and layered closure is performed. A Jones compressive dressing, along with a posterior splint, is applied. Sutures or staples are removed in the office at 2 weeks.

The patient is maintained in a splint for the initial 2 weeks and then transitioned to cast or posterior splint for the next 4 to 6 weeks. Nonweightbearing status is maintained throughout this period until consolidation of fracture is identified. When consolidation of the fracture is observed on radiographs, the patient will be transitioned to partial weightbearing in a controlled ankle motion (CAM) walker boot.

COMPLICATIONS

Complications that can arise specific to the technique of MIPO for distal tibia fracture include medial ankle wound complications, painful prominent hardware, and iatrogenic damage to the greater saphenous vein and saphenous nerve.

Ozsoy and colleagues[9] reported their results from a cadaveric study evaluating risk of injury to the saphenous nerve and the greater saphenous vein with the MIPO technique for distal tibia fractures. They reported a high risk of injury to both the saphenous nerve and the greater saphenous vein with percutaneous screw placement using distal tibia locking compression plates. They advocate careful dissection and protection of the soft tissue for percutaneous screw placement.

Prominence of the hardware with associated skin irritation or impingement is another common complication reported. Lau and colleagues[10] reported skin impingement in 52% of their patients treated by MIPO. Those patients eventually had their hardware removed. With advancements in fracture fixation, plates are evolving into more low profile plates. This may aid in reducing hardware prominence and skin impingement.

DISCUSSION

Treatment of distal tibia fractures with articular involvement can be a very arduous task. This type of injury often creates a predicament for the surgeon. There are various techniques and approaches to surgically treat distal tibia fractures, including IMN, external fixation, ORIF, and MIPO. Each type of fixation has its own advantages and disadvantages. The difficult decision lies in which fixation option will create the most structurally stable environment along with best return of function, keeping in mind minimizing risk of complications.

IMN performed in an antegrade fashion for treatment of distal tibia fractures has been associated with a high rate of knee morbidity. Studies have reported chronic anterior knee pain among the more common complications. The cause is unclear and may be due to the disruption and iatrogenic injury to the patellar tendon and associated soft tissue structures.[11] Toivanen and colleagues[12] reported on chronic anterior knee pain after antegrade IMN of distal tibia fractures in 67% of their patients at final follow-up, with most of those patients being mildly to severely impaired by the pain.

Fracture malalignment has also been reported with use of intramedullary nails. In a randomized, prospective comparison study of IMN versus plate osteosynthesis performed by Vallier and colleagues,[4] they found similar union rates between the 2 groups. They did report an increased rate of 23% malalignment with use of IMN compared with plating. Beytemur and colleagues[13] reported on a comparison study between IMN and MIPO for AO-OTA type 43 C1-C2 distal tibia fractures. They found similar results with time to union, functional scores, and complications. One facet of their results that they noted was the increased presence of valgus malunions in the IMN group.

Biomechanical factors also play a significant role in fixation choice, especially with plate fixation of unstable fractures. Optimal plate fixation should contain the strength and stability afforded by the implant to withstand external forces and to protect the fracture during the time needed for osseous consolidation. Yenna and colleagues[8] evaluated the biomechanical properties of medial plates and anterolateral plates for distal tibia fractures. Evaluation of plate stiffness in both axial and torsional loading was performed with sawbone models, which were created to represent AO-OTA type 43 A2 fractures. They found that there was no significant difference in stiffness between the medial and anterolateral plate constructs with application of external compression or torsional forces.

The incision used for ORIF of distal tibia fractures requires extensive dissection of the soft tissue. This has been noted to lead to poor healing and increased wound complications. Incisions made over the anterior ankle have been shown to compromise the angiosome of the anterior tibial artery. In their anatomic study evaluating the anterolateral incision, Fisher and colleagues[14] reported that an average of 9.3 perforating

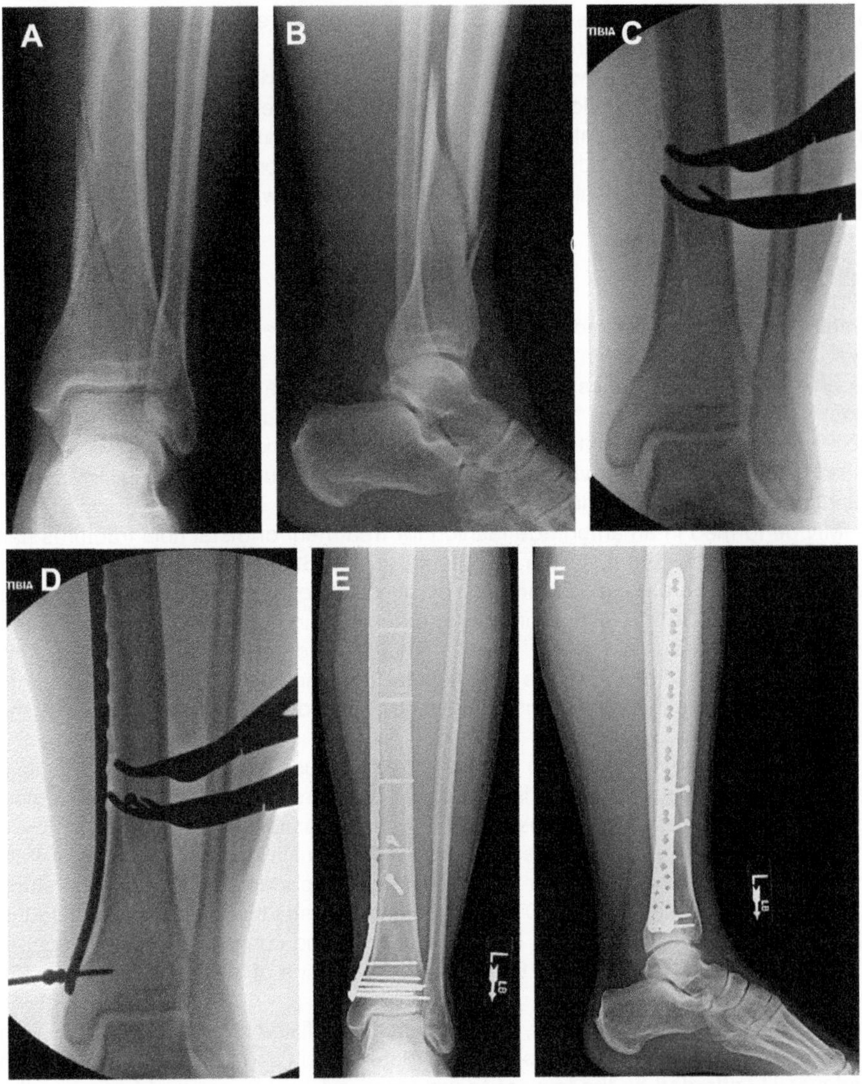

Fig. 4. (*A*) AP radiograph of a distal tibia fracture. (*B*) Lateral radiograph of a distal tibia fracture. (*C*) Fluoroscopy used to aid in fracture reduction of distal tibia fracture with bone clamps. (*D*) Fluoroscopic image displaying placement and temporary fixation of the medial distal tibia plate. (*E*) AP radiograph displaying complete consolidation of a distal tibia fracture via MIPO technique. (*F*) Lateral radiograph displaying complete consolidation of a distal tibia fracture via MIPO technique.

vessels were encountered and were at increased risk for injury. They concluded that there was a high risk for iatrogenic wound complications from creation of this incision. Borrelli and colleagues[7] performed a study evaluating vascular supply to the distal tibia and found that open plating compared with percutaneous plating significantly disrupted the extraosseous blood supply. Open plating prevented periosteal vessels from filling and functioning properly. They concluded that this correlates with poor healing of the wound, as well as the fracture site, and may ultimately require further intervention if healing is not obtained. The anterolateral incision has an increased morbidity with high rates of wound complications, which has been well-documented in the literature. Bhattacharyya and colleagues[15] reported wound complications of 32%, with one-half developing deep infection when ORIF was performed through a posterolateral approach. These results were similar to the wound complications reported for other incisional approaches for ORIF of distal tibia fractures. The development of wound complications after surgical treatment is of severe gravity because it may result in exposure of the tibia, as well as the hardware, owing to the limited surrounding soft tissue, which may be catastrophic.

MIPO for distal tibia fractures has been reported in the literature to have favorable outcomes. Results of high union rates and decreased instances of malalignment have been noted with use of MIPO for distal tibia fractures (**Fig. 4**). Functional outcomes and decreased wound complications have also been reported in the literature.[16,17] Collinge and colleagues[16] reported a 92% union rate with good to excellent functional outcomes in treatment of distal tibia fractures with MIPO. Ahmad and colleagues[17] discussed their positive results of functional outcomes with an average American Orthopedic Foot and Ankle Society Score (AOFAS) ankle score of 88.8. They also noted union in 16 of 17 patients at an average of 23.1 weeks (union at 15.3 weeks in nonsmokers and 32 weeks in smokers). Similar results were reported in a prospective study performed by Paluvadi and colleagues.[18] They reported an average time to union at 21.4 weeks and excellent functional outcomes with an average AOFAS score of 95.06.

MIPO for distal tibia fractures is a treatment option that has proven to have great overall results. It provides substantial structural stability, along with respect to the soft tissue envelope and vascular supply, compared with other fixation methods. MIPO is a valuable method for treatment of distal tibia fractures that provides a high rate of union and return to function, along with decreased wound complications.

REFERENCES

1. Thordarson D. Complications after treatment of tibial pilon fractures: prevention and management strategies. J Am Acad Orthop Surg 2000;8:253–65.
2. Teeny S, Wiss D. Open reduction and internal fixation of tibial plafond fractures. Variables contributing to poor results and complications. Clin Orthop Relat Res 1993;292:108–17.
3. Dillin L, Slabaugh P. Delayed wound healing, infection and nonunion following open reduction and internal fixation of tibial plafond fractures. J Trauma 1986; 26(12):1116–9.
4. Vallier H, Cureton B, Patterson B. Randomized, prospective comparison of plate versus intramedullary nail fixation for distal tibia shaft fractures. J Orthop Trauma 2011;25(12):736–41.
5. Lefaivre K, Guy P, Chan H. Long-term follow-up of tibial shaft fractures treated with intramedullary nailing. J Orthop Trauma 2008;22:525–9.

6. Encinas-Ullan C, Fernandez-Fernandez R, Rubio-Suarez J, et al. Medial versus lateral plating in distal tibial fractures: a prospective study of 40 fractures. Rev Esp Cir Ortop Traumatol 2013;57(2):117–22.
7. Borrelli J, Prickett W, Song E, et al. Extraosseous blood supply of the tibia and the effects of different plating techniques: a human cadaveric study. J Orthop Trauma 2002;16(10):691–5.
8. Yenna Z, Bhadra A, Ojike N, et al. Anterolateral and medial locking plate stiffness in distal tibial fracture model. Foot Ankle Int 2011;32(6):630–7.
9. Ozsoy M, Tuccar E, Demiryurek D, et al. Minimally invasive plating of the distal tibia: do we really sacrifice saphenous vein and nerve? A cadaveric study. J Orthop Trauma 2009;23:132–8.
10. Lau T, Leung F, Chan C, et al. Wound complication of minimally invasive plate osteosynthesis in distal tibia fractures. Int Orthop 2008;32(5):697–703.
11. Jankovic A, Korac Z, Bozic N, et al. Influence of knee flexion and atraumatic mobilisation of infrapatellar fat pad on incidence and severity of anterior knee pain after tibial nailing. Injury 2013;44:33–9.
12. Toivanen J, Valsto O, Kannus P, et al. Anterior knee pain after intramedullary nailing of fractures of the tibial shaft. A prospective, randomized study comparing two different nail-insertion techniques. J Bone Joint Surg Am 2002;84-A(4):580–5.
13. Beytemur O, Baris A, Albay C, et al. Comparison of intramedullary nailing and minimal invasive plate osteosynthesis in the treatment of simple intra-articular fractures of the distal tibia (AO-OTA type 43 C1-C2). Acta Orthop Traumatol Turc 2017;51(1):12–6.
14. Fisher B, Nathan S, Acland R, et al. The anterolateral incision for pilon fracture surgery: an anatomic study of cutaneous blood supply. Acta Orthop Belg 2011;77:355–61.
15. Bhattacharyya T, Crichlow R, Gobezie R, et al. Complications associated with the posterolateral approach for pilon fractures. J Orthop Trauma 2006;20:104–7.
16. Collinge C, Protzman R. Outcomes of minimally invasive plate osteosynthesis for metaphyseal distal tibia fractures. J Orthop Trauma 2010;24:24–9.
17. Ahmad M, Sivaraman A, Zia A, et al. Percutaneous locking plates for fractures of the distal tibia: our experience and a review of the literature. J Trauma 2012;72(2):81–7.
18. Paluvadi S, Lal H, Mittal D, et al. Management of fractures of the distal third tibia by minimally invasive plate osteosynthesis - a prospective series of 50 patients. J Clin Orthop Trauma 2014;5(3):129–36.

Primary Arthrodesis in Severely Comminuted Fractures

Michael W. Downey, DPM[a,*], Ted C. Lai, DPM[b,1], Justin J. Fleming, DPM[c]

KEYWORDS

• Comminuted fractures • Primary fusion • Arthrodesis • Intra-articular fracture • High-energy trauma

KEY POINTS

- Severely comminuted fractures of the foot and ankle are caused by high-energy trauma.
- Adhering to proper lower extremity trauma protocol on initial examination is of utmost importance in order to address emergent situations and to prevent development of major sequelae.
- Understanding the morphology and biomechanics of the affected joint aids in the decision making of performing primary arthrodesis in the lower extremity for successful outcomes.
- Primary fusion of severely comminuted fractures provides predictable outcomes with less chance of developing posttraumatic arthritis and need for revisional surgery.

INTRODUCTION

Arthrodesis remains the gold standard for resolution of painful recalcitrant joints with osteoarthritis in the foot and ankle. Controversy regarding the appropriate treatment of complex injuries exists. Coetzee and Ly[1] supported primary fusion of the tarsometatarsal (TMT) joint for Lisfranc fracture-dislocation rather than open reduction and internal fixation (ORIF) in instances of severe ligamentous injury as well as articular comminution.[1] Sanders and colleagues[2] showed the benefit of fusion of the subtalar joint (STJ) in the presence of a multifragmented comminution injury (type 4) to the calcaneus affecting the posterior facet.[2] Advances in literature and fusion techniques

Disclosure: The authors have nothing to disclose.
[a] Trinity Foot & Ankle Specialists, 5801 Oakbend Trail #140, Fort Worth, TX 76132, USA; [b] Shore Orthopaedic University Associates, 24 MacArthur Boulevard, Somers Point, NJ 08244, USA; [c] University Orthopaedic Associates, 2 World's Fair Drive, Somerset, NJ 08873, USA
[1] Present address: 205 Cambridge Avenue, Linwood, NJ 08221.
* Corresponding author.
E-mail address: Michael.W.Downey@gmail.com

Clin Podiatr Med Surg 35 (2018) 233–257
https://doi.org/10.1016/j.cpm.2017.12.006
podiatric.theclinics.com

provide confidence for functional and satisfactory outcomes for these injuries. The literature is sparse for primary arthrodesis in the setting of severe traumatic articular damage to the ankle, talonavicular (TN), calcaneocuboid (CC), naviculocuneiform (NC), and first metatarsophalangeal (MTP) joints. This article challenges the threshold of decision for primary fusion in the setting of severely comminuted fractures.

Treatment plans can become fulminant when the injuries are associated with high-energy trauma affecting the articular surface. When approaching any fracture, the main priority is to correct deformity and mitigate posttraumatic arthritis. Intra-articular fractures can be elusive, leading to severe morbidity. As the degree of comminution and injury to the articular surface increases, obtaining near-perfect anatomic alignment of the joint surface becomes an indirectly proportional task. Even when anatomic alignment is achieved, chances of developing posttraumatic arthritis are high. Cartilage impaction and involvement with ankle fractures has been reported up to 79% to 90%, ultimately leading to an increased prevalence of poorer outcomes.[3,4]

Management of high-energy foot and ankle injuries continues to be a challenge. Even with near-perfect anatomic reduction by experienced surgeons, recovery is poor and posttraumatic arthritis is substantially increased.[5–7] Further complications can ensue with primary ORIF to include specific patient demographics, wound dehiscence, malunion/depression of fragments, osteonecrosis, limb shortening, shortened columns of the foot, and continued pain, all leading to meager patient satisfaction.

Although literature is sparse and inconclusive, surgeon preference typically dictates the use of primary fusion for resolution of traumatic foot and ankle injuries affecting the chondral surface. Although primary fusion should be used under specific indications, this article further adds to the literature detailing successful and predictable outcomes in primary arthrodesis to eliminate the high probability of posttraumatic arthritis, obviates additional operations secondary to arthritic development or other complications, and improves long-term functional outcomes.

EVALUATION AND WORK-UP

On initial evaluation, proper trauma assessment of the patient is an absolute. Once stabilized, a proper history and physical helps determine the nature of the injury, which aides in the treatment plan. A thorough history, including comorbidities and social history, is important for the treatment plan. Advanced comorbidities, such as uncontrolled diabetes mellitus, end-stage renal disease, vascular or neurologic deficits, as well as tobacco or drug abuse, should guide the surgeon to a more aggressive treatment plan in approaching unstable intra-articular fracture patterns.

Physical examination requires a complete evaluation of bilateral lower extremities. Severe trauma to one extremity often masks other existing index injuries that the patient may not be able to properly report. Lower extremity focused examination should start proximally in evaluating the proximal tibia and fibular head then progressing distally to examination of all tendinous structures of the foot and ankle, simultaneously assessing the neurovascular status. High suspicion of compartment syndrome and symptoms associated with the sequelae is necessary. Other emergent and/or high-suspicion situations of lower extremity trauma include neurovascular compromise, open fractures, and compromise to the soft tissue from skin tenting.

Radiographic imaging aids in diagnosis of the injury and gives details on the severity of the fractures. Obtaining contralateral images is often beneficial in differentiating pathologic findings from normal host variants.

Other imaging modalities that are necessary in this setting for both diagnosis as well as surgical preparation include computed tomography (CT) scan. CT scans provide an in depth three-dimensional (3D) view of the fracture and the joint involved. Along with 3D reconstruction of the CT scan, the surgeon can appreciate the amount of comminution, impactions, die punch fragments, chondral step-offs, and malalignments. When CT scans are obtained, the surgeon should direct how the CT scan is to be performed. CT scans with 1.25-mm slices reoriented to the affected joint are helpful, if available, to determine the appropriate assessment of chondral injury.

MRI and ultrasonography are also useful imaging modalities for the foot and ankle but have less impact on surgical planning for primary fusion of complex fractures. These imaging modalities are better used for evaluation of associated soft tissue injuries.

INITIAL TREATMENT

After a thorough examination has been completed, initial restoration and suitable alignment of the fracture and adjacent joints are necessary to assist severe dislocations of the foot and ankle, which leads to damage of surrounding soft tissue structures, the soft tissue envelope, and neurovascular compromise.

Closed reduction can be done in the emergency room setting under a local block or conscious sedation followed by splintage for maintenance of reduction. There are instances in which closed reduction under conscious sedation cannot be obtained, in which the patient may require full sedation in the operating suite for closed reduction or application of a spanning external fixator.

Other considerations with high-energy trauma of the foot and ankle are open fractures and compartment syndrome. With open fractures, it is necessary to start the patient on intravenous (IV) antibiotics. Timing of administration of IV antibiotics has been reported in the literature as one of the major factors in decreasing chance of infection. IV antibiotics are to be administered within 1 hour of injury. Antibiotics are to be selected based on the Gustilo-Anderson classification for open fractures. Grade 1 is treated with a first-generation cephalosporin, grade 2 with a first-generation cephalosporin and aminoglycoside, and grade 3 with the addition of penicillin for anaerobes.[8] The fracture is then taken to the operating room for debridement and possible stabilization with external fixator pending instability.

Compartment syndrome is another emergent condition in which diagnosis is made by clinical assessment and confirmed with intracompartmental pressures. Once confirmed, an emergent fasciotomy of the foot or leg should be performed.

Maintaining anatomic reduction with high-energy injuries is often difficult because of inherent instability of the fracture. These injuries may require temporary fixation with percutaneous pinning and/or application of a spanning external fixator. The use of external fixation aids in bringing the fracture out to length, maintaining anatomic reduction, and preventing subsidence and soft tissue compromise.

Spanning external fixators can be fashioned in many different forms, ranging from delta frames for ankle and pilon fractures to monorail frames for medial or lateral column injuries of the foot. The stabilization of the fracture with the use of external fixation allows for the soft tissue envelope to stabilize and swelling to subside in preparation for definitive treatment.

INDICATIONS

Primary fusion for fractures of the foot and ankle should be reserved for high-energy trauma and complex fractures. The major indication for primary fusion is severe comminution of the articular surface. The joint may present with severe impaction deformity, delaminated cartilage, or high-grade comminution. These types of injuries make attempts at restoring the articular surface to its anatomic alignment futile. These aspects of intra-articular fractures have been reported to cause progressive development of posttraumatic arthritis even when proper restoration of the articular surface is obtained. Additional factors directing toward primary fusion in this trauma setting include difficult social circumstances and/or severe noncompliance. These factors may increase the risk of complications resulting in posttraumatic arthritis and ultimately requiring additional procedures in the future.

Forefoot Primary Fusion

First metatarsophalangeal joint fractures

Metatarsal fractures are fairly common and usually occur at the midshaft. They are typically treated with standard ORIF and have been noted to have successful outcomes. Nevertheless, intra-articular fractures to the MTP joints are often difficult to manage. The injury is usually caused by direct trauma or crush injuries, which often result in open fractures or severe comminution. When comminuted fractures are present to the first MTP joint, primary fusion has been noted to be a viable treatment option.

Comminuted fractures to the first MTP joint frequently result in a severe soft tissue zone of injury along with associated shortening of the first ray. Spanning external fixation in the form of a monorail can be used to pull the first ray out to length and prevent soft tissue contracture.

- Primary fusion of the first MTP joint is performed with a dorsal linear incision over the first MTP joint.
- The extensor hallucis longus tendon is examined at this area to identify an injury to the tendon.
- The tendon is retracted laterally to gain exposure to the first MTP joint fracture.
- The spanning external fixator can be used to further distract the joint for better exposure.
- Larger fracture fragments are reduced and temporarily fixated with Kirschner wires (k-wires).
- The articular surface of the fracture fragments of the first metatarsal head and proximal phalanx base are debrided down to healthy bleeding subchondral bone.
- Because of the high grade of comminution, osseous defects are often present.
- Autogenous bone graft from the calcaneus or distal tibia can be harvested and used to fill the defect and bridge the gap to prevent significant shortening.
- Fixation depends on surgeon preference; however, locking plates offer adequate stability for primary fusion of the first MTP joint.
- For severely comminuted unstable fractures to the first MTP joint, double plating may be used, in which plates are positioned on both the dorsal and medial aspects of the fusion site.
- This construct provides added stability to the fusion (**Fig. 1**).

Fusion of the first MTP joint has been shown in the literature to have successful outcomes.[9] DeFrino and colleagues[9] performed a prospective study on first MTP joint fusion for hallux rigidus, and they reported effective pain relief with excellent patient satisfaction.[9] Functional outcomes were noted to improve with an American Orthopaedic Foot & Ankle Society (AOFAS) score of 38 preoperatively to 90 postoperatively.[9] Brodsky and colleagues[10] evaluated functional outcomes of first MTP joint fusions.[10] The investigators reported an average pain score of 11 on the visual

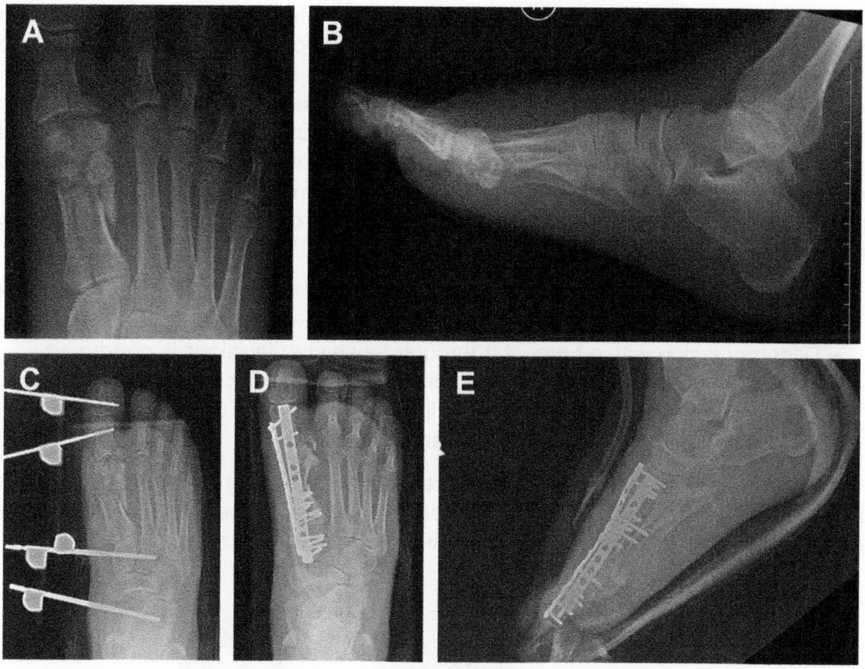

Fig. 1. (*A*) Anteroposterior (AP) radiograph of comminuted first MTP joint. (*B*) Lateral radiograph of comminuted first MTP joint. (*C*) Spanning external fixation is applied to provide stability to the first ray. (*D*) AP radiograph showing primary fusion of the first MTP joint with double plating technique. Fixation is extending proximally to address the first TMT joint. (*E*) Lateral radiograph showing primary fusion of the first MTP joint with double plating technique. Fixation is extending proximally to address the first TMT joint.

analogue scale of 100.[10] In addition, they found positive results with a 94% satisfaction rate, 98% return to preoperative occupation without any restrictions, and most of the patients being able to return to recreational activities.[10] Although the successful outcomes were from studies involving first MTP joint fusion as treatment of degenerative joint disease, comparisons can be made for success with a primary fusion as well. Primary fusion of the first MTP joint for traumatic complex fractures involves a more severe cause compared with degenerative joint disease; however, outside the zone of injury and possible soft tissue complications, the fixation constructs are similar. Fusion of the first MTP joint provides pain relief, deformity correction, and also creates stability of the first ray during ambulation.

Tarsometatarsal Primary Fusion

Tarsometatarsal joint fractures

High-energy trauma to the Lisfranc complex often leads to complete disruption of the TMT joint. This condition can occur from falls from heights, direct trauma, or motor vehicle accidents, which have been observed in about 40% to 45% of cases.[11] This high-energy trauma to the Lisfranc joint often results in high-grade comminution of the TMT joint, dislocation, and/or complete instability of the ligamentous structures. At present, controversy regarding the appropriate treatment of complex Lisfranc injuries exists. Coetzee and Ly[1] supported primary fusion of the TMT joint for Lisfranc fracture-dislocation rather than ORIF in instances of severe ligamentous injury as well as articular comminution. Studies have shown favorable results following primary fusion of purely ligamentous and comminuted fractures of the Lisfranc joint.[1]

On initial evaluation, emergent situations are assessed. Fasciotomies for Lisfranc fractures are performed to decompress the interosseous, medial, lateral, and central compartments. This procedure had traditionally been performed with 2 large incisions on the dorsum of the foot (**Fig. 2**). These large fasciotomies often delay definitive surgical correction because of the time required for healing of these wounds. Pie-crusting fasciotomy is a more forgiving, less invasive technique.[12]

- This procedure entails making rows of 1-cm linear incisions along the dorsum of the foot along each interosseous compartment.
- Decompression with a hemostat through these stab incisions is performed.
- The stab incisions heal quickly with a formation of an eschar over the incision.
- The incisions for definitive Lisfranc primary fusion can be made directly over the previously created row of stab incisions (**Fig. 3**).

After initial evaluation is complete and treatment of restoring anatomic reduction is obtained, radiographic imaging and CT scans are reviewed. The soft tissue swelling is given adequate time to resolve before definitive surgical treatment.

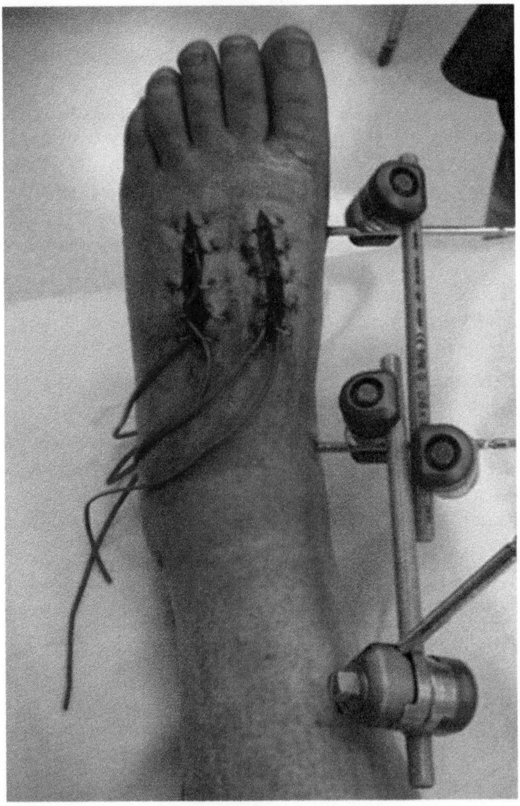

Fig. 2. Dual-incision fasciotomies are performed on the dorsum of the foot. Dorsomedial and dorsolateral incisions decompress the interosseous, central, medial, and lateral compartments. Shoelace technique is performed to aid in gradual closure of these large incisions.

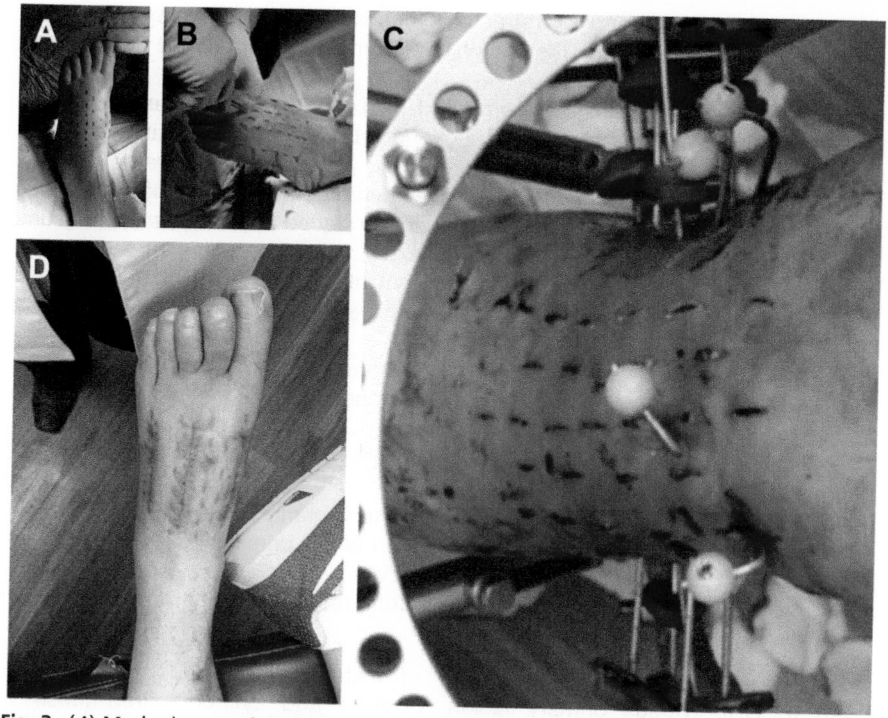

Fig. 3. (*A*) Marked-out stab incisions on the dorsum of the foot for pie-crusting fasciotomy. (*B*) Decompression of the compartments is performed with a hemostat through the stab incisions. (*C*) Early healing of the pie-crusting fasciotomy is noted with scab formation over the stab incisions. (*D*) Healed incisions from the pie-crusting fasciotomy and primary fusion of the TMT joint. Primary fusion incisions were made directly over the row of previously made stab incisions.

Fusion is typically performed on the first, second, and third TMT joints and is not advised for the fourth and fifth TMT joints because of the degrees of motion necessary for biomechanical transition from midstance to toe-off. In a cadaveric study by Ouzounian and Shereff,[13] minimal motion to the medial and middle columns and significant motion of the lateral column were noted. The first TMT joint showed 3.5° of motion, the second and third TMT joints had 0.6° to 1.6° of motion, and the fourth and fifth TMT joints had 9.6° to 10.2° of motion. Conclusions were made that the medial and middle columns had minimal motion with no significant loss noted after fusion of these joints.

Incision placement is determined on the fracture pattern and the necessary aspects of fusion over these joints. The incision placements used are the same as are used for ORIF.

- Medial incision is made over the first TMT joint. Dorsal linear incisions are made over the interval between the first and second TMT joints and an additional dorsal incision over the third TMT joint.
- Meticulous dissection is made through the fascia with care being taken to avoid the branches from the medial and intermediate dorsal cutaneous nerves.
- Incision is made through the capsule of the first, second, and third TMT joints, giving exposure to the joint surfaces.

- A Hintermann retractor or pin retractor is then placed on the metatarsal base and corresponding cuneiform. Distraction is performed to open up the comminuted TMT joint.
- Preparation of the joint is then performed, with curettes, osteotomes, and a burr used to remove the cartilage and subchondral bone, with copious irrigation over the burr to prevent thermal necrosis.
- Once all the joints are completely debrided and prepared, bone graft, cancellous allograft cubes, biologics, and so forth can be placed at the fusion site.
- The forefoot is grasped and a dorsiflexory force is placed on the foot to create compression and proper alignment of the TMT joint for fusion. With the position held stable, 1.6-mm k-wires are used to temporarily fixate the TMT joint.
- Fixation can then be performed with 3.5-mm fully threaded screws placed from the dorsal metatarsal base to the corresponding cuneiform when applicable (**Fig. 4**). With highly comminuted fractures, plate fixation is mostly likely to be the choice of fixation; 3.5-mm locking straight or T-plates for fusion of the Lisfranc joint can be used (**Fig. 5**).
- The fourth and fifth TMT joints are then temporarily fixated with 0.062-mm k-wires percutaneously. The lateral column is not primarily fused because of the amount of motion needed to be preserved.
- Closure is performed in layered fashion. Compression dressings and a posterior splint are applied.

Controversy still exists for treatment of high-energy Lisfranc injuries with regard to ORIF versus primary fusion. Coetzee and Ly[1] compared these 2 types of surgical treatments for Lisfranc fractures. Their results were significantly favorable for primary fusion compared with ORIF. AOFAS midfoot scores of 88 were noted for the primary fusion group compared with 68.6 for the ORIF group.[1] They also noticed patients in the primary fusion group reported an estimated 92% return to preinjury activity level compared with 65% in the ORIF group.[1] Coetzee and Ly[1] concluded that primary fusion should be indicated for Lisfranc fractures with either purely ligamentous disruption with multiplanar instability of severe comminution to the joint.[1] Henning and colleagues[14] compared primary arthrodesis versus ORIF for Lisfranc fractures and found no significant differences in function with regard to the Short Form-36 (SF-36) or short musculoskeletal functional assessment (SMFA) scores.[14] They did note significant results for secondary surgeries, which included hardware removal and revisional arthrodesis, in which 16.7% of the primary arthrodesis group required secondary surgeries compared with 78.6% in the ORIF group.[14] Primary arthrodesis for highly comminuted or purely ligamentous Lisfranc fractures have shown favorable results with regard to function, decreased complications, and decreased need for additional procedures.

Midfoot Primary Fusion (Navicular, Cuneiforms, Cuboid)

Highly comminuted fractures of the midfoot, to include the navicular, cuboid, and cuneiforms, can be insidious. Although uncommon, they are usually associated with a high-energy proximal Lisfranc variant and/or impaction. Loss of length of the medial and lateral columns is observed when significant comminution is present in the navicular or cuboid respectively. Initial management and length restoration of these associated columns becomes an important factor to restore the contiguous anatomy.

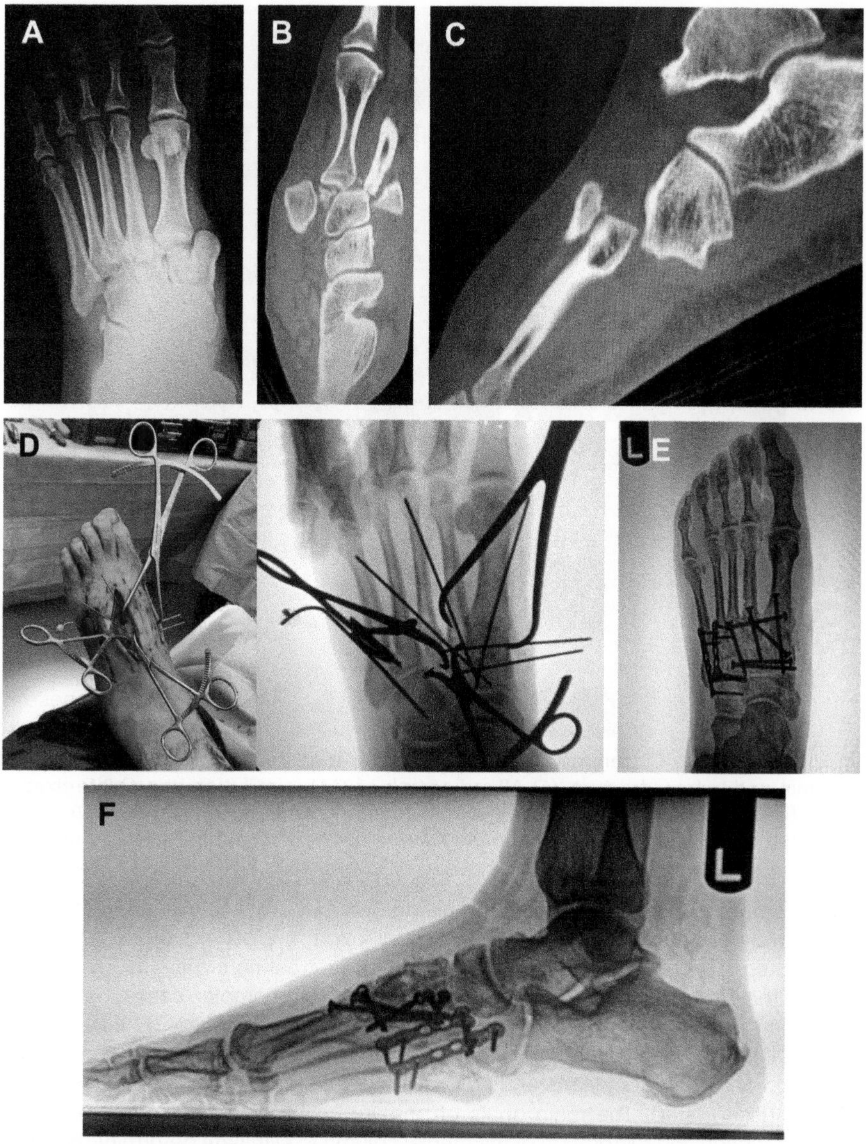

Fig. 4. (*A*) AP radiograph of a Lisfranc fracture-dislocation. (*B*) Axial-view CT scan showing comminuted medial column of the TMT joint. (*C*) Sagittal-view CT scan showing complete dislocation of the TMT joint lateral column. (*D*) Intraoperative reduction and fusion of the TMT joint. (*E*) AP radiograph of primary fusion of the TMT joint using screw fixation. Bridge plating is used for the lateral column. (*F*) Lateral radiograph of primary fusion of the TMT joint using screw fixation. Bridge plating is used for the lateral column.

Cuneiform/navicular fractures

High-energy trauma affecting the navicular typically results in severe comminution and/or fracture-dislocation. The mechanism is a direct source or an axial compression insult as a Lisfranc proximal variant. Sangeorzan and colleagues[15] classified navicular body fractures into 3 types. Type 1 is a transverse body fracture with a low-energy

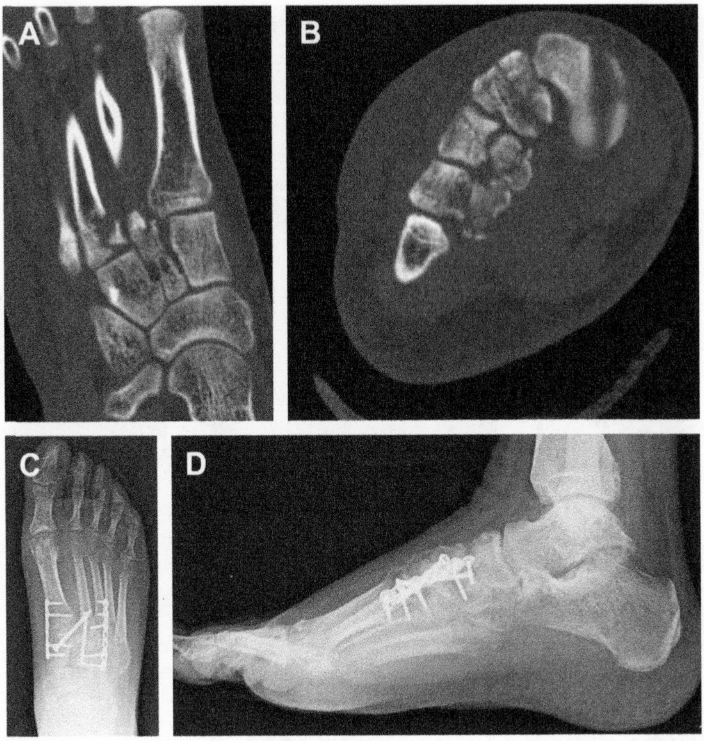

Fig. 5. (*A*) Axial-view CT scan of a comminuted Lisfranc fracture. (*B*) Coronal-view CT scan of a comminuted Lisfranc fracture. (*C*) AP radiograph of TMT joint fusion using plate fixation on the first and third TMT joints. The lateral column was previously pinned. (*D*) Lateral radiograph of TMT joint fusion using plate fixation on the first and third TMT joints.

mechanism, type 2 is a dorsomedial to plantar lateral body fracture, and type 3 is a central body fracture along with lateral comminution.[15] When encountering severe comminuted navicular and adjacent joint structures, treatment may involve primary fusion of the TN joint, naviculocuneiform joint, or, in more complex cases, medial column fusion involving all of these joints. Primary arthrodesis of the TN joint is often reserved if the surgeon is able to spare this joint fusion because it controls the remaining motion of the hindfoot joints and acts as a medium throughout the biomechanical gait (discussed later). The main goals of primary fusion for navicular fractures are proper reduction and restoration of the medial column to eliminate deformity/malalignment, prevent long-term sequelae, and create a pain-free plantigrade gait; and maintaining the integrity of the surrounding soft tissue with special attention to avoiding damage to the posterior tibial tendon.[16] With evaluating the osseous injury along with surgical planning, it is also important to take into consideration the vascular supply to the navicular, because it has robust extraosseous blood supply compared with its limited intraosseous blood supply.[17] Theoretically, primarily fusing the navicular to the cuneiforms can provide increased vascularization of the comminuted navicular.[16]

- Primary fusion of the medial column can be done with a single or double incision. The single medial utility incision is carried over the dorsomedial aspect.
- The 2-incision approach is performed on the medial aspect of the midfoot and over the central aspect of the dorsum of the foot to gain access and exposure

to the lateral TN and naviculocuneiform joints. One complication of the single-incision approach is not having adequate exposure of the lateral aspect of the medial column, resulting in the inability to obtain proper joint preparation and consequently developing nonunion. This complication can be mitigated with an incision directed slightly more dorsal just medial to the anterior tibial tendon if the soft tissue envelope and zone of injury allows. With the double-incisional approach, there is concern for vascular disruption to the navicular.[15]
- Once access is gained into the TN and/or naviculocuneiform joints, exposure is obtained with use of Hintermann retractors.
- Joint preparation is performed with use of curettes, osteotomes, and/or burr.
- Copious irrigation is used with the burr to prevent thermal necrosis of the fusion site.
- Meticulous joint preparation is performed with care to preserve the structural contour of these joints.
- Before fixation, the joints may be augmented with bone graft or biologic substitutes.
- There are some instances in which comminution of the navicular is such that severe bone loss is present. In this scenario, autogenic or allogenic bone grafting can be used to restore shape to the navicular and bring the medial column back to length.
- Temporary fixation is performed with 1.6-mm k-wires. Goals of positioning and reduction are restoring the length of the medial column with the appropriate metatarsal declination angle addressed.
- Fixation for primary fusion involving the navicular is based on surgeon preference. Fixation choices can range from 3.5-mm fully threaded lag screws, anatomic plates, and compression plates. Decisions for fixation should address columnar alignment, being careful to avoid irritation from surrounding soft tissue structures as well as not affecting the medial or lateral aspects of the associated fractures (**Fig. 6**).
- Medial column fusion plates are also available for TN, NC, and first TMT joints. Compression is difficult with these plates, even with the eccentric drill holes; nevertheless, restoration of columns and alignment of the joints with added biologics for augmentation as well as mild deficits from bone loss is imperative compared with aggressive compression.

Complications of concern for primary fusion of joints associated with navicular fractures are adjacent joint arthritis, malunion, nonunion, avascular necrosis, and posterior tibial tendon disruption.

Cuboid fracture

Fractures are elusive and even more uncommonly observed as isolated fractures. Fractures to the cuboid are often accompanied by Lisfranc caused by lateral impaction or direct crushing injuries. The fracture pattern usually results in impaction and depression of the articular surfaces. Lateral impaction cuboid fractures are often described as nutcracker fractures because of the longitudinal compression of the cuboid where it sits between the calcaneus and the fourth and fifth metatarsal when axial forces are applied to the lateral column.[18] The comminution involved with cuboid fractures typically results in collapse and shortening of the lateral column.

On initial examination, it is necessary to determine whether lateral column length is present. Obtaining contralateral radiographs to evaluate and compare may identify even a subtle loss in length. CT scan is a more useful imaging modality along with

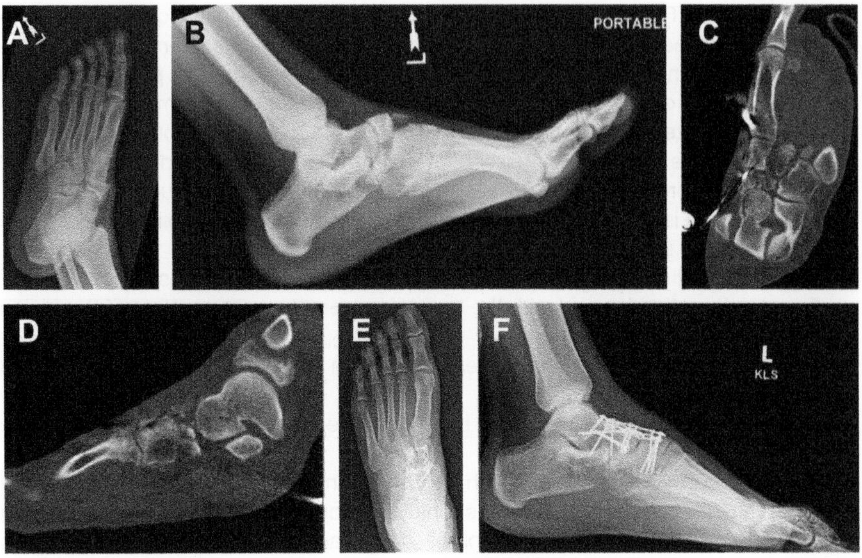

Fig. 6. (*A*) Medial oblique radiograph displaying comminuted fracture of the lateral navicular. (*B*) Lateral radiograph of comminuted navicular fracture-dislocation. (*C*) CT scan axial view of comminuted lateral navicular. (*D*) CT scan sagittal view of comminuted navicular. (*E*) Medial oblique radiograph of primary TN joint fusion. (*F*) Lateral radiograph showing fusion of the TN joint with plate fixation spanning the NC joint.

use of CT 3D reconstruction, because it aids in visualization and appreciation of the fracture pattern as well as in noting loss of length.

If lateral length loss is observed, a spanning mini–external fixator can be applied to span the fracture and bring the soft tissue component out to length to avoid contracture. Once the soft tissue swelling has subsided, definitive surgery is performed.

ORIF can be performed if significant articular comminution is not involved. The impacted distal and/or proximal articular surface can be disimpacted or elevated with gentle manipulation, temporarily fixated with a k-wire, and cancellous allograft or autograft packing can be obtained to restore relative anatomic shape. This process is then followed by screw and plate fixation.[19] There are several plating systems that are made to fit the contour of the cuboid for fracture repair.

Significant comminution to the articular surfaces creates a more complex repair. When the distal articular surface is comminuted, primary fusion of the cuboid to the fourth and fifth metatarsal can result in poor outcomes caused by locking the motion of the necessary lateral TMT joint complex for an advantageous biomechanical gait.

- Comminuted fractures to the proximal articular surface of the cuboid can be treated with primary fusion of the CC joint.
- The incision is made on the dorsolateral aspect of the cuboid and is extended proximally past the CC joint.
- Care is taken to identify and gently retract/protect the sural nerve.
- If initial temporary distraction with a spanning monorail external fixator is not performed and lateral column shortening is noted with definitive fixation, a spanning external fixator can be used in conjunction with the fusion to bring the lateral column out to length. This technique avoids complications with soft tissue contracture.

- The external fixation device can stay during the healing process in order to provide minute adjustments if necessary throughout the fusion postoperative period.
- When addressing the impacted articular surface, the dorsolateral wall of the cuboid must first be elevated to gain access to the depressed fragments.
- Restoration of length can be performed by elevating the depressed proximal articular surface with a freer elevator or a small osteotome.
- The remaining articular surface of the cuboid and the anterior calcaneal process are debrided with the use of curettes, osteotomes, and/or burr.
- Copious irrigation is used with the burr to prevent thermal necrosis of the fusion site.
- Allograft or autograft can be used to pack the osseous defect. It is important to use an adequate amount of graft to bring the lateral column completely out to length to avoid malalignment or compensation-type pain caused by inadequate length.
- Fixation is then performed with 2.7-mm and 3.5-mm screws and/or plate fixation.

The main goal of primary fusion of the comminuted cuboid fracture is to restore lateral column length because failure to do this can lead to significant deformity and disability. Shortening of the lateral column produces an abduction deformity of the forefoot, which creates compensation in the form of a pes planovalgus deformity (**Fig. 7**).[18]

Complications observed include malunion, nonunion, posttraumatic arthritis, lateral column collapse, shortening (which may result in development of flat foot deformity), and sural nerve injury.

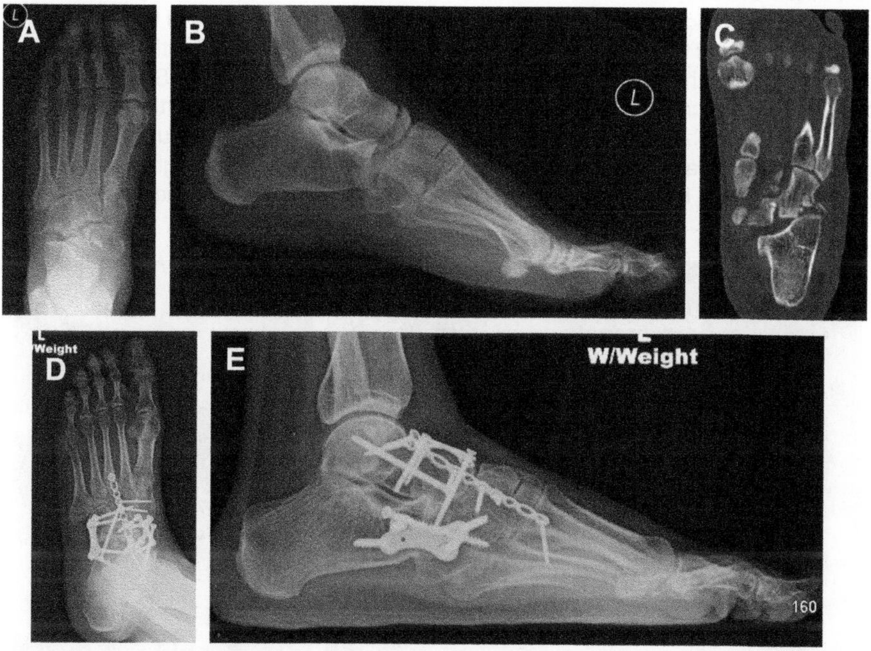

Fig. 7. (*A*) AP radiograph of a comminuted proximal cuboid fracture. Comminution is also noted at the lateral navicular body. (*B*) Lateral radiograph displaying comminuted cuboid and navicular fracture. (*C*) Axial CT scan showing impaction and comminution of the proximal lateral cuboid. (*D*) Medial oblique radiograph of primary fusion of the CC and TN joints. (*E*) Lateral radiograph showing complete consolidation of the CC and TN joints.

Rearfoot Primary Fusion

Calcaneal fractures

When approaching high-energy fracture patterns to the calcaneus, the prognosis is poor and these can be life-altering injuries for these patients. ORIF is the mainstay of surgical repair for intra-articular calcaneal fractures but this has been reported in the literature to show less favorable results in the highly comminuted Sanders type 3 and type 4 fractures. Primary arthrodesis has been suggested as a preferable treatment, with convincing outcomes for Sanders type 4 calcaneal fractures.[20]

On initial evaluation, it is necessary to rule out compartment syndrome for these high-energy fracture patterns. If diagnosed with compartment syndrome, appropriate intervention must be performed for decompression of the compartment. The sequelae of compartment syndrome include functional impairment to both musculature and nervous system. There are also reports of worsening outcomes with associated calcaneal fractures compared with calcaneal fractures without compartment syndrome.[21] These investigators showed AOFAS scores of 52 for patients diagnosed with calcaneal fractures and missed compartment syndrome compared with 77.4 for patients with calcaneal fractures without compartment syndrome symptoms.[21] The approach is directed on the medial calcaneus 1 cm above the glabrous border and linearly directly anterior to the tubercle. Layer-by-layer dissection over the abductor hallucis is recommended as the septum is approached, being careful to avoid neurovascular injury in the process of releasing the calcaneal compartment (**Fig. 8**).

There may also be situations in which comminuted calcaneal fractures require closed reduction or pinning in the initial phases followed by the appropriate time for soft tissue swelling to subside. Cases in which the STJ is significantly impacted or the tuber is significantly shortened may be treated with initial external fixation to bring the calcaneus out to length. This procedure can also be performed with percutaneous screw fixation with the push-screw technique for indirect reduction. Schildhauer and colleagues[22] described this procedure for severely depressed intra-articular calcaneal fractures for which definitive surgery must be delayed.[22] This procedure is performed by drilling and placement of a fully threaded 6.5-mm screw through the calcaneal tuber. The screw is advanced across the calcaneal body toward the posterior talar

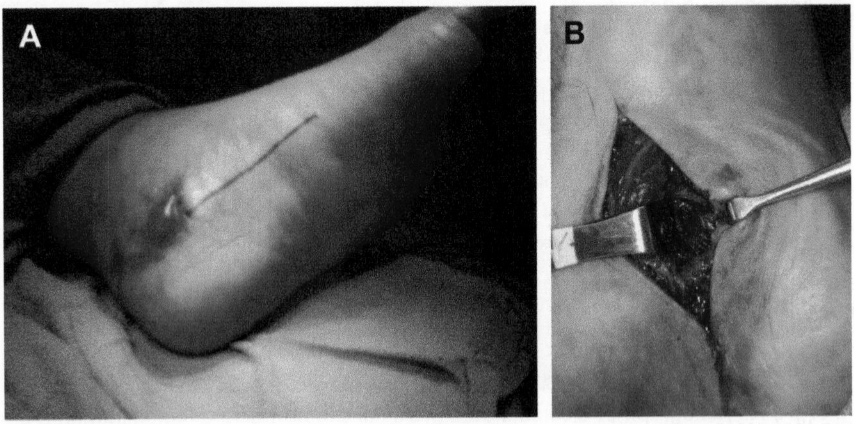

Fig. 8. (*A*) Fasciotomy of the calcaneal compartment is performed on the medial calcaneus 1 cm above the glabrous border. (*B*) Decompression of the medial and calcaneal compartment is performed. The increased compartment pressure causes herniation of the abductor hallucis muscle belly.

body with special attention not to advance through the posterior face of the talus. This push screw is then used to indirectly reduce the depressed calcaneal fracture by pushing against the talar posterior facet, which in turn pushes the tuber posteriorly and brings the calcaneal tuberosity out to length. An additional 6.5-mm screw is then inserted across the STJ into the talus to hold this correction out to length. This technique reestablishes the calcaneal height and length initially to allow for the soft tissue swelling to subside for delayed primary fusion.[22]

Surgical approach for primary STJ fusion for severely comminuted intra-articular fractures can be performed with 2 different approaches: the lateral extensile and the sinus tarsi approaches. The sinus tarsi incision is used more often because it has less inherent risk with regard to postoperative wound complications.

- The sinus tarsi approach is a linear oblique incision made on the lateral aspect of the rear foot centered directly over the posterior facet. This incision is made from the distal tip of the fibula extending to the fourth metatarsal base.
- Dissection is carried deeper, with care taken to identify and gently retract the peroneal tendons inferiorly. Exposure to the lateral STJ is then achieved.
- The depressed fracture fragments are then elevated with use of a Freer elevator or similar instrument.
- Fracture reduction along with realignment of the calcaneal tuber is then performed, at which time a Schanz pin is then inserted into the lateral aspect of the posterior calcaneal tuber laterally to medially.
- The Schanz pin is then used as a joystick to aid in reduction of the fracture, in which the tuber is brought out to length, rotated out of varus, and restoration of the Bohler angle is achieved. Reduction is performed to realign the medial calcaneal wall back to the sustentaculum, which is observed under fluoroscopy or digital radiographs to confirm proper anatomic reduction in all 3 planes and then temporarily fixated with 0.062 k-wires or smaller Steinmann pins.
- Once reduction is achieved, the STJ is then prepared for primary fusion.
- Removal of cartilage and subchondral bone is performed with the use of curettes, osteotomes, and/or burr.
- Copious irrigation is used with the burr to prevent thermal necrosis of the fusion site.
- Any osseous defects are packed with cancellous cubes.
- The fusion site can be augmented with bone graft or biologic grafts.
- Fixation for the primary STJ fusion is then performed based on the surgeon preference of large fully or partially threaded cannulated screws. Usually 2 and sometimes 3 screws (if necessary) are inserted from the posterior inferior aspect of the calcaneal tuberosity and advanced across the prepared STJ.
- Screws are positioned with one being in the talar body and the other in the talar neck and head region (**Fig. 9**).

Restoring articular congruity, height, width, and normal anatomic shape of the calcaneus results in improved patient satisfaction and long-term results.[23] Use of primary ORIF in severely comminuted intra-articular calcaneal fractures has proved difficult, with further development of STJ arthrosis and poor hindfoot function.[20,24–26] These outcomes may lead to an arthrodesis despite attempts to fixate in an optimal position, because hindfoot motion becomes limited.[20,24–27] There have been suggestions that restoring morphology is more important than anatomic congruity because of the limited motion at the STJ.[23,28–30] The incidence of primary arthrodesis has increased because of greater complication rates in higher energy fractures.[20,24] These complications include soft tissue compromise, loss of reduction, and severe

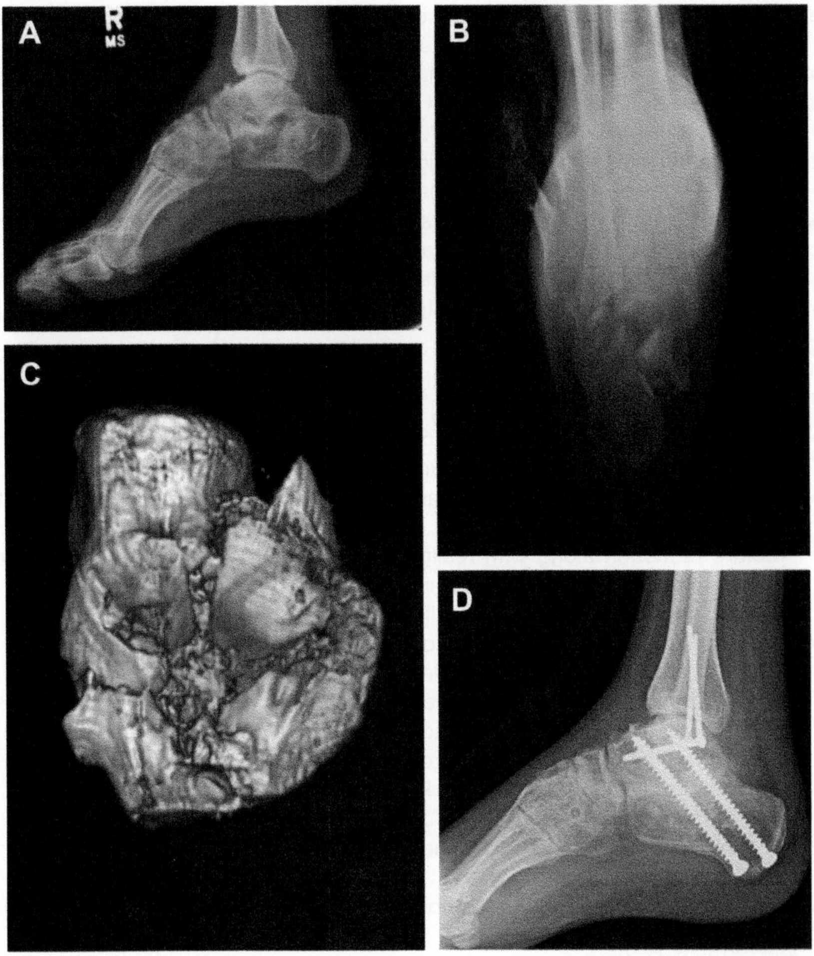

Fig. 9. (*A*) Lateral radiograph displaying a severely comminuted intra-articular calcaneal fracture. (*B*) Calcaneal axial radiograph displaying a severely comminuted intra-articular calcaneal fracture. (*C*) CT 3D reconstruction of the comminuted articular surface of the calcaneus. (*D*) Primary arthrodesis of the STJ using fully threaded screws. ORIF of the medial malleolus and talar body was also performed.

posttraumatic arthritis, even with excellent intraoperative reduction.[31] Allmacher and colleagues[32] relate that even patients who show spontaneous fusion report more favorable outcomes than those with preservation of STJ motion.[32] Radnay and colleagues[23] related that operative intervention and restoration of the morphology of the calcaneus results in better long-term functional outcomes for patients who eventually went onto an STJ arthrodesis.[23] Holm and colleagues[33] studied primary fusion for comminuted fractures of the calcaneus and showed favorable outcomes after the procedure, especially when the radiographic relationships of the hindfoot were restored.[33] These investigators reported AOFAS hindfoot scores of 78, with the maximum possible being 94.[33] They related that even better outcomes were shown when patient age was considered.[33] An STJ incision is preferred rather than an extended lateral incision because of soft tissue compromise over the lateral flap.[34]

The lateral extensile is at times necessary for restoration of height and width; however, it is an absolute contraindication in patients without the lateral calcaneal branch of the peroneal artery.[35] Bibbo and colleagues[35] showed 100% wound dehiscence when the artery was absent for lateral extensile incisions.[35] Timing is normally dictated by the soft tissue envelope and delay in intervention, which does not create a more difficult approach for primary fusion.

Talar fractures

Talus fractures are often amenable to ORIF. However, in cases with severe comminution to the posterior facet of the STJ, primary fusion becomes a viable treatment option. Surgical correction and restoration of the articular surface become daunting tasks because of the fracture pattern as well as persistent high rates of posttraumatic arthritic formation. Primary fusion can offer a better alternative to restore the anatomic structure to the rear foot along with prevention of predictable posttraumatic arthritis to eliminate further surgical needs (discussed earlier).

Depending on the fracture location and type, primary fusion can be approached with talar head fractures, neck fractures, body fractures, or fractures affecting the posterior facet. Whether TN fusion, STJ fusion, or ankle joint fusion are needed, proper anatomic reduction is of utmost importance because of reestablishment of the vasculature as well as prevention of nonunion and/or malunion.

Fractures or fracture-dislocations involving the TN joint make anatomic reduction difficult. A hyperdorsiflexory force at the ankle joint with inversion puts this important midtarsal joint at risk, subsequently resulting in a comminuted neck fracture and possible talar head subluxation/dislocation (type 4).[36,37] Compressive loading through the sustentaculum tali with a crush injury or an axial load through the navicular with a shear injury can affect the navicular body or talar head directly.[38] A proximal variant Lisfranc injury with an axial force through the metatarsals can indirectly affect the TN joint (discussed earlier). There is an association between the prognosis and the severity of injury at the TN joint with the degree of initial displacement.[39] With severe impaction or comminution at the TN joint, the remaining talus and/or the cuneiforms may be used as a template for reconstruction and limit disorder at the adjacent midtarsal joint or midfoot joints.[39] Additional surgery may be avoided for increasing posttraumatic arthritis in the medial column. Johnstone and Maffulli[40] relate that primary fusion of a severely fractured navicular bone can be used to restore medial column length and eliminate complications associated with increasing posttraumatic arthritis and malunion.[40] Earlier reports have advocated primary TN joint fusion in cases of severe comminution; however, when these reports were published, there was limited evidence supporting this treatment option in high-energy fractures.[41–44] Thomas and Daniels[45] showed a successful TN and STJ primary arthrodesis for a type 4, nonreconstructable, severely comminuted talar neck fracture with talar head extension with ankle joint motion restored.[45] They relate that a delay in presentation prompted them toward fusion; however, many reports relate that type 4 talar neck fractures result in inauspicious outcomes.[36,46,47]

Soft tissue compromise can delay the window for primary repair initially. Contracture of adjacent soft tissue as well as substantial chondral wear can create difficulty in reduction and anatomic repair. Marked displacement, fracture blisters, and ischemic skin caused by tension from underlying bone prompt an urgent reduction with either a spanning external fixator, wire fixation, bioabsorbable repair, or internal fixation device.

Fracture repair with internal fixation can have limitations caused by the initial soft tissue compromise and extensive comminution. Subacute or chronic avascular necrosis after fixation of the proximal Lisfranc variant, the navicular, or talar head/neck can create changes dynamically leading to impaction of the medial column, acquired flat foot changes, and a more difficult and demanding late-stage reconstruction with poor patient satisfaction.

The talus is covered in up to 60% of hyaline articular cartilage, which leaves a limited surface area for blood supply.[48] It has been well documented that the talar head and neck are supplied by the dorsalis pedis artery and anastomosis from the peroneal arteries, whereas the talar body is supplied inferiorly by the tarsal canal and sinus tarsi arteries, and superiorly the talar body is supplied by the deltoid artery.[49] The blood supplies acts as a sling around the talus and further complications ensue when these structures are disrupted secondary to traumatic injury. Osteonecrosis of the talar body has been reported in up to 100% with type 4 talar neck fractures.[36,46,50] Despite this outcome, several level IV studies have indicated that the risk of osteonecrosis can be reduced with anatomic reduction and stable internal fixation.[36,46,51,52] Lindvall and colleagues[53] relate unions in as many as 88% with open fixation.[53] With such a high percentage for union and a concomitantly high rate of osteonecrosis, it can deduced that fusion or additional surgeries are likely even with near anatomic reduction for fracture repair. Vallier and colleagues[54] reported results of open repair of 60 talar neck fractures and the effect of the surgical delay compared with osteonecrosis and found no correlation between the timing of fixation and development of osteonecrosis.[54] However, they did note that there was a worsening prognosis of osteonecrosis associated with high-energy talar neck injuries,[54] making primary fusion an advantageous option initially. High-energy talar body fractures pose similar difficulties in fracture care and complications. These fractures can be approached with concepts and principles similar to those of ankle primary fusion. The same principles apply for ankle primary fusion.

Ankle Primary Fusion

Pilon/tibia plafond fractures

High-energy fractures to the distal tibia and tibial plafond create severe osseous and soft tissue zones of injuries. Initial evaluation for these injuries begins with the rule-out of compartment syndrome, evaluating any open fractures and/or soft tissue defects, and confirming an intact neurovascular status. These emergent situations are limb threatening and should be addressed immediately. LeBus and Collinge[55] reported on vascular injuries resulting from high-energy pilon fractures. These investigators report that, through the use of CT angiography, 52% of their patients had anomalies to the vasculature of their distal leg.[55] Of this 52% with vascular injury, 69% involved the anterior tibial artery (**Fig. 10**).[55]

Following initial evaluation, staging of the pilon fracture is performed. In the first stage, spanning external fixation is applied for temporary structural stabilization. Distal fibular fractures can be addressed during the staging with ORIF. However, if primary fusion is an option, this decision may need to be delayed. CT scans are typically ordered after stabilization of these fracture patterns for detailed assessment and surgical planning.

- Primary fusion of the ankle joint has been described with multiple surgical approaches, including lateral, anterior, posterior, and arthroscopic.
- It has also been described with various techniques, including external fixation, intramedullary nailing, and ORIF.
- With severely comminuted pilon fractures, either an anterior or lateral approach is performed with the use of a tibiotalocalcaneal intramedullary nail.

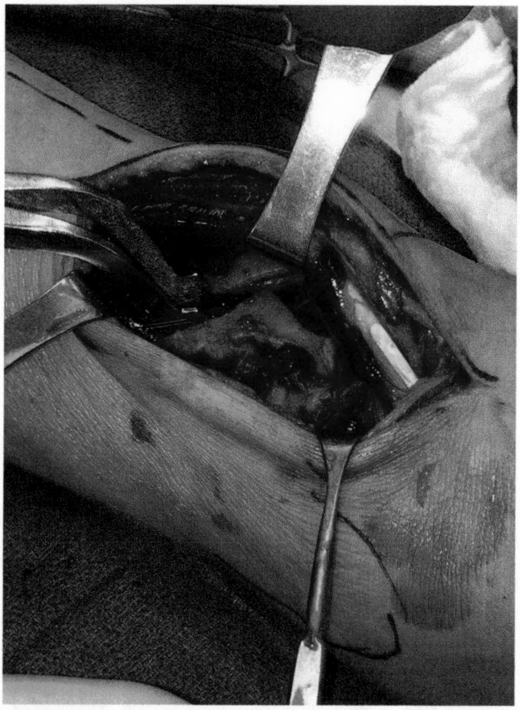

Fig. 10. Highly comminuted distal tibia fracture with neurovascular bundle entrapment.

- In the anterior approach, the delta frame external fixator is left in place because this aids in joint distraction and manipulation of the fracture.
  - An incision is made in the midline of the ankle.
  - Dissection is deepened through the subcutaneous layer.
  - The surgical interval is made between the tibialis anterior tendon and extensor hallucis longus tendon.
  - The tibialis anterior tendon is retracted medially and the extensor hallucis longus tendon, along with the neurovascular bundle and adjacent lateral tendons, is retracted laterally.
- The anterior aspect of the comminuted tibia plafond is exposed.
  - The fracture fragments are anatomically reduced to maintain length and alignment.
  - Smaller comminuted fragments and die-punch fragments may be removed because they will be replaced later with bone graft.
  - The articular surface from fracture fragments of the tibial plafond is debrided of its cartilage.
  - The cartilage of the talar dome is also debrided down to healthy subchondral bleeding bone.
  - A 2.0-mm drill bit is suggested to fenestrate the talus and tibial plafond.
  - Osseous defects of the distal tibia are then backfilled with autogenous or allogeneic bone graft.
  - Orthobiologics may also be used to augment fusion of the ankle joint.
  - Appropriate apposition of the tibiotalar joint is performed and temporarily fixated with pins or k-wires.

- Fixation is then performed with either an anterior ankle fusion plate or retrograde intramedullary nail.
  - Retrograde intramedullary nailing may better span the zone of injury than plate fixation.
  - Plating can also be used in conjunction to intramedullary nailing to aid in reduction of larger fracture fragments of the distal tibia (**Fig. 11**).
- For the lateral transfibular approach, the spanning external fixator is left in place for distraction of the joint.
  - The lateral rod from the delta frame is removed to create better exposure.
  - The incision is made on the lateral aspect of the distal leg extending down to the lateral STJ.
  - The peroneal musculature is retracted posteriorly and dissection is made down to the fibula.

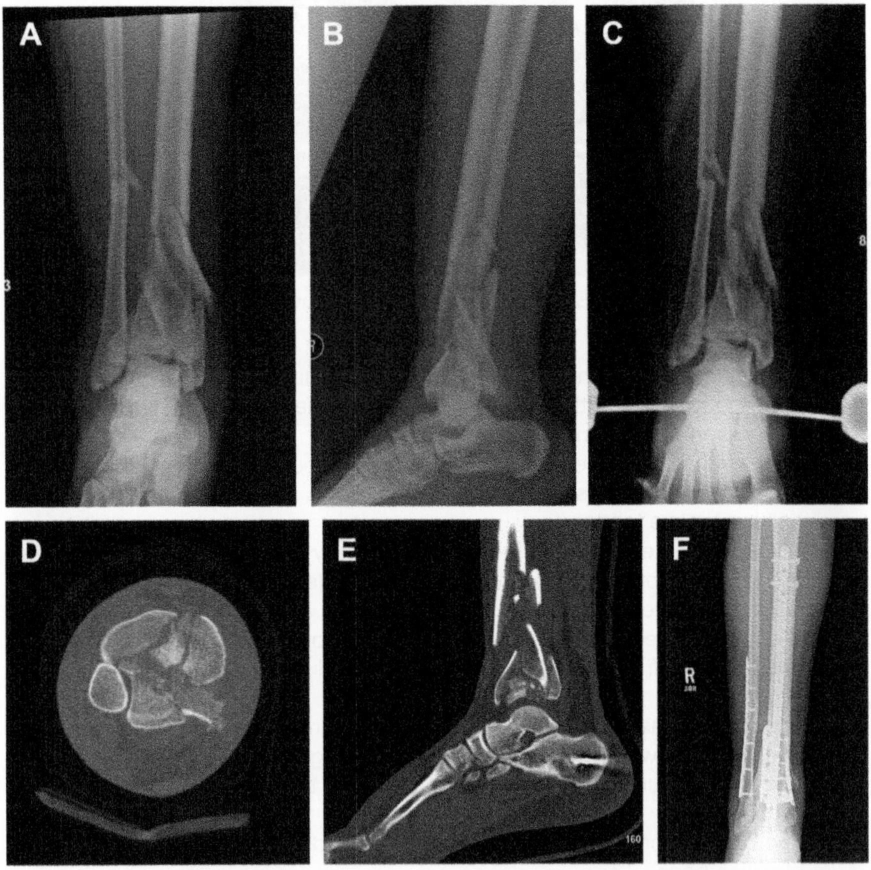

Fig. 11. (*A*) AP radiograph of AO/OTA 43-C3 pilon fracture. (*B*) Lateral radiograph of AO/OTA 43-C3 pilon fracture. (*C*) AP radiograph after reduction with application of delta external fixator. (*D*) CT axial view displaying comminuted tibial plafond. (*E*) CT sagittal view displaying comminuted tibial plafond fracture. (*F*) AP radiograph after primary ankle fusion with a retrograde intramedullary nail. Distal tibia anterolateral plate and medial buttress plate were used in addition for reduction of the larger distal tibia fracture fragments. Complete consolidation is noted.

  - The distal fibula is then transected at the distal one-third level and removed, giving exposure to the lateral ankle and STJ.
  - Fracture fragments are reduced and the articular surface is debrided of its cartilage from both the plafond and talus.
- The STJ is also addressed from this incision.
  - Dissection is carried down to the lateral STJ.
  - The articular surface is then debrided of its cartilage to the level of subchondral bleeding bone.
  - Primary fusion of the ankle through the lateral approach is then fixated with either a lateral plate that spans the tibiotalocalcaneal joints or with an intramedullary nail.

Pilon or tibial plafond fractures are typically performed in a staged fashion.[56,57] Blauth and colleagues[58] showed that a 2-stage procedure had greater ankle range of motion, decreased pain, and improved return to work.[58] Despite a bulky external fixation device and possible pin-tract infections, this mainstay approach suggests improved patient outcomes for lower energy AO/OTA type A and B pilon fractures.[5,6,58] However, functional long-term results remain poor for higher energy AO/OTA type C fractures.[5,59] Pollak and colleagues[60] looked at patients scoring with high-energy pilons as well as some patients who had AO/OTA type B pilon fractures and compared those scores with known values from other studies that documented scoring with medical comorbidities.[60] They showed that the SF-36 scores for these fractures are less than the SF-36 scores of patients with multiple traumatic injuries, pelvic fractures, diabetes mellitus, acute myocardial infarction, and acquired immunodeficiency syndrome.[60] Patient demographics may also be attributed to outcome factors; Pollak and colleagues[60] showed poorer scores and outcome measures for patients with 2 or more comorbidities, who were married, who had an annual income of less than $25,000, and patients who were without a high-school diploma.[60] The investigators conclude that patients with these injuries have worse scores than age-matched and gender-matched norms.[60] Harris and colleagues[5] showed a 31% and 69% incidence of posttraumatic arthritis for pilons repaired with either ORIF or circular ring external fixation respectively and related that AO/OTA type C pilon fractures have an increased risk for developing posttraumatic arthritis.[5] Marsh and colleagues[6] related a significant decrease in SF-36 score for pilon fractures and a 70% incidence of tibiotalar arthritis with patients treated with an external fixator and/or ORIF at a 5-year to 11-year follow-up.[6] Malunion of the plafond surface has been reported in as many as 70%[58] and continues to be problematic with subsidence and developing osteonecrosis.[5] Wound complications have been reported in as many as 37% for surgical reduction with an open procedure for pilon fractures because soft tissue management of pilon repairs has been known to be one of the biggest challenges.[56,61] Infection after an ORIF can further complicate the initial repair, leading to septic fusion and even amputation.[5,61,62] Zelle and colleagues[63] compared a posterior blade plate arthrodesis performed primarily with high-energy pilon fractures and related that their results were equivalent or higher on 3 of 8 SF-36 subscales for the primary fusion group.[63] They concluded that the functional status was favorable and supported a primary fusion for these fracture types.[63] Further, they had no wound complications, which they attribute to their posterior approach, and all patients walked without support of a cane, walker, or crutches.[63] Hsu and colleagues[64] relate that early ankle arthrodesis with a tibiotalocalcaneal intramedullary retrograde nail can be reserved for severely comminuted fractures, impacted fragility fractures, obese diabetic patients, fractures with poor bone quality, or patients in resource-limited environments who refuse to comply with protocols.[64] In addition, these investigators report that high-risk patients requiring early stability and weight bearing may be better suited for primary arthrodesis with an intramedullary tibiotalocalcaneal retrograde nail, with the advantage of decreased soft tissue dissection and decreased implant bulk compared with pilon plates.[64] Bozic and colleagues[59] reported 15 nonreconstructable pilon fractures that were treated with primary fusion and showed excellent results, with all 15 patients showing stable fusion at 15 weeks and independent ambulation at 39 weeks.[59] Niikura and colleagues[65] evaluated 2 patients with comminuted pilon fractures that they deemed nonreconstructable and that were treated with an antegrade intramedullary nail from the proximal tibia.[65] The investigators related that both patients could ambulate independently and were pain free at 1 year or greater follow-ups.[65]

SUMMARY

Management of high-energy foot and ankle fractures can be difficult. Indications for primary fusion of high-energy foot and ankle injuries should take into account patient selection, realistic long-term functional goals, and avoiding subsequent returns to the operating theater for revision surgery secondary to a complication with initial ORIF or subsequent arthrodesis caused by posttraumatic arthritis. Each treatment should be tailored to severe articular comminution, the amount of bone loss, limited/poor socioeconomic factors, and ultimately the needs of each patient. Primary fusion is a viable treatment option and provides a potentially advantageous alternative in approaching these challenges. The present article extrapolates successful literature-based reports of foot and ankle fusions and extends the suggestion of primary fusion for high-energy/traumatic foot and ankle injuries for improved long-term outcomes. Further, the present article adds to the limited existing body of literature regarding outcomes in primary arthrodesis for these associated foot and ankle injuries.

REFERENCES

1. Coetzee JC, Ly TV. Treatment of primarily ligamentous Lisfranc joint injuries: primary arthrodesis compared with open reduction and internal fixation. Surgical technique. J Bone Joint Surg Am 2007;89(Suppl 2 Pt.1):122–7.
2. Sanders R, Fortin P, DiPasquale T, et al. Operative treatment in 120 displaced intraarticular calcaneal fractures. Results using a prognostic computed tomography scan classification. Clin Orthop Relat Res 1993;(290):87–95.
3. Thomas B, Yeo JM, Slater GL. Chronic pain after ankle fracture: an arthroscopic assessment case series. Foot Ankle Int 2005;26(12):1012–6.
4. Hintermann B, Regazzoni P, Lampert C, et al. Arthroscopic findings in acute fractures of the ankle. J Bone Joint Surg Br 2000;82(3):345–51.
5. Harris AM, Patterson BM, Sontich JK, et al. Results and outcomes after operative treatment of high-energy tibial plafond fractures. Foot Ankle Int 2006;27(4):256–65.
6. Marsh JL, Weigel DP, Dirschl DR. Tibial plafond fractures. How do these ankles function over time? J Bone Joint Surg Am 2003;85-A(2):287–95.
7. Wyrsch B, McFerran MA, McAndrew M, et al. Operative treatment of fractures of the tibial plafond. A randomized, prospective study. J Bone Joint Surg Am 1996;78(11):1646–57.
8. Gustilo RB, Anderson JT. Prevention of infection in the treatment of one thousand and twenty-five open fractures of long bones: retrospective and prospective analyses. J Bone Joint Surg Am 1976;58(4):453–8.

9. DeFrino PF, Brodsky JW, Pollo FE, et al. First metatarsophalangeal arthrodesis: a clinical, pedobarographic and gait analysis study. Foot Ankle Int 2002;23(6):496–502.
10. Brodsky JW, Passmore RN, Pollo FE, et al. Functional outcome of arthrodesis of the first metatarsophalangeal joint using parallel screw fixation. Foot Ankle Int 2005;26(2):140–6.
11. Nunley JA, Vertullo CJ. Classification, investigation, and management of midfoot sprains: Lisfranc injuries in the athlete. Am J Sports Med 2002;30(6):871–8.
12. Dunbar RP, Taitsman LA, Sangeorzan BJ, et al. Technique tip: use of "pie crusting" of the dorsal skin in severe foot injury. Foot Ankle Int 2007;28(7):851–3.
13. Ouzounian TJ, Shereff MJ. In vitro determination of midfoot motion. Foot Ankle 1989;10(3):140–6.
14. Henning JA, Jones CB, Sietsema DL, et al. Open reduction internal fixation versus primary arthrodesis for Lisfranc injuries: a prospective randomized study. Foot Ankle Int 2009;30(10):913–22.
15. Sangeorzan BJ, Benirschke SK, Mosca V, et al. Displaced intra-articular fractures of the tarsal navicular. J Bone Joint Surg Am 1989;71(10):1504–10.
16. DiGiovanni CW. Fractures of the navicular. Foot Ankle Clin 2004;9(1):25–63.
17. McKeon KE, McCormick JJ, Johnson JE, et al. Intraosseous and extraosseous arterial anatomy of the adult navicular. Foot Ankle Int 2012;33(10):857–61.
18. Borrelli J Jr, De S, VanPelt M. Fracture of the cuboid. J Am Acad Orthop Surg 2012;20(7):472–7.
19. Sangeorzan BJ, Swiontkowski MF. Displaced fractures of the cuboid. J Bone Joint Surg Br 1990;72(3):376–8.
20. Sanders R, Lindvall E. Fractures and fracture-dislocations of the talus. In: Coughlin MJ, Mann R, Saltzman CL, editors. Surgery of the foot and ankle. 8th edition. Philadelphia: Mosby; 2007. p. 2075–136.
21. Rosenthal R, Tenenbaum S, Thein R, et al. Sequelae of underdiagnosed foot compartment syndrome after calcaneal fractures. J Foot Ankle Surg 2013;52(2):158–61.
22. Schildhauer TA, Sangeorzan BJ. Push screw for indirect reduction of severe joint depression-type calcaneal fractures. J Orthop Trauma 2002;16(6):422–4.
23. Radnay CS, Clare MP, Sanders RW. Subtalar fusion after displaced intra-articular calcaneal fractures: does initial operative treatment matter? J Bone Joint Surg Am 2009;91(3):541–6.
24. Schepers T. The primary arthrodesis for severely comminuted intra-articular fractures of the calcaneus: a systematic review. Foot Ankle Surg 2012;18(2):84–8.
25. Thermann H, Hufner T, Schratt E, et al. Long-term results of subtalar fusions after operative versus nonoperative treatment of os calcis fractures. Foot Ankle Int 1999;20(7):408–16.
26. Hetsroni I, Nyska M, Ben-Sira D, et al. Analysis of foot and ankle kinematics after operative reduction of high-grade intra-articular fractures of the calcaneus. J Trauma 2011;70(5):1234–40.
27. Bozkurt M, Kentel BB, Yavuzer G, et al. Functional evaluation of intraarticular severely comminuted fractures of the calcaneus with gait analysis. J Foot Ankle Surg 2004;43(6):374–9.
28. Buckley R, Tough S, McCormack R, et al. Operative compared with nonoperative treatment of displaced intra-articular calcaneal fractures: a prospective, randomized, controlled multicenter trial. J Bone Joint Surg Am 2002;84-A(10):1733–44.
29. Rammelt S, Amlang M, Barthel S, et al. Percutaneous treatment of less severe intraarticular calcaneal fractures. Clin Orthop Relat Res 2010;468(4):983–90.

30. Schuberth JM, Cobb MD, Talarico RH. Minimally invasive arthroscopic-assisted reduction with percutaneous fixation in the management of intra-articular calcaneal fractures: a review of 24 cases. J Foot Ankle Surg 2009;48(3):315–22.
31. Howard JL, Buckley R, McCormack R, et al. Complications following management of displaced intra-articular calcaneal fractures: a prospective randomized trial comparing open reduction internal fixation with nonoperative management. J Orthop Trauma 2003;17(4):241–9.
32. Allmacher DH, Galles KS, Marsh JL. Intra-articular calcaneal fractures treated nonoperatively and followed sequentially for 2 decades. J Orthop Trauma 2006;20(7):464–9.
33. Holm JL, Laxson SE, Schuberth JM. Primary subtalar joint arthrodesis for comminuted fractures of the calcaneus. J Foot Ankle Surg 2015;54(1):61–5.
34. Kline AJ, Anderson RB, Davis WH, et al. Minimally invasive technique versus an extensile lateral approach for intra-articular calcaneal fractures. Foot Ankle Int 2013;34(6):773–80.
35. Bibbo C, Ehrlich DA, Nguyen HM, et al. Low wound complication rates for the lateral extensile approach for calcaneal ORIF when the lateral calcaneal artery is patent. Foot Ankle Int 2014;35(7):650–6.
36. Daniels TR, Smith JW. Talar neck fractures. Foot Ankle Int 1993;14(4):225–34.
37. Sneppen O, Buhl O. Fracture of the talus: a study of its genesis and morphology based upon cases with associated ankle fracture. Acta Orthop Scand 1974;45(1–4):307–20.
38. Ahmad J, Raikin SM. Current concepts review: talar fractures. Foot Ankle Int 2006;27(6):475–82.
39. Main BJ, Jowett RL. Injuries of the midtarsal joint. J Bone Joint Surg Br 1975;57(1):89–97.
40. Johnstone AJ, Maffulli N. Primary fusion of the talonavicular joint after fracture dislocation of the navicular bone. J Trauma Acute Care Surg 1998;45(6):1100–2.
41. Coltart WD. Aviator's astragalus. J Bone Joint Surg Br 1952;34-B(4):545–66.
42. Early JS. Management of fractures of the talus: body and head regions. Foot Ankle Clin 2004;9(4):709–22.
43. Pennal GF. Fractures of the talus. Clin Orthop Relat Res 1963;30:53–63.
44. Thordarson DB. Talar body fractures. Orthop Clin North Am 2001;32(1):65–77, viii.
45. Thomas RH, Daniels TR. Primary fusion as salvage following talar neck fracture: a case report. Foot Ankle Int 2003;24(4):368–71.
46. Canale ST, Kelly FB Jr. Fractures of the neck of the talus. Long-term evaluation of seventy-one cases. J Bone Joint Surg Am 1978;60(2):143–56.
47. Pajenda G, Vecsei V, Reddy B, et al. Treatment of talar neck fractures: clinical results of 50 patients. J Foot Ankle Surg 2000;39(6):365–75.
48. Rammelt S, Zwipp H. Talar neck and body fractures. Injury 2009;40(2):120–35.
49. Weston JT, Liu X, Wandtke ME, et al. A systematic review of total dislocation of the talus. Orthop Surg 2015;7(2):97–101.
50. Comfort TH, Behrens F, Gaither DW, et al. Long-term results of displaced talar neck fractures. Clin Orthop Relat Res 1985;(199):81–7.
51. Archdeacon M, Wilber R. Fractures of the talar neck. Orthop Clin North Am 2002;33(1):247–62, x.
52. Berlet GC, Lee TH, Massa EG. Talar neck fractures. Orthop Clin North Am 2001;32(1):53–64.
53. Lindvall E, Haidukewych G, DiPasquale T, et al. Open reduction and stable fixation of isolated, displaced talar neck and body fractures. J Bone Joint Surg Am 2004;86(10):2229–34.

54. Vallier HA, Reichard SG, Boyd AJ, et al. A new look at the Hawkins classification for talar neck fractures: which features of injury and treatment are predictive of osteonecrosis? J Bone Joint Surg Am 2014;96(3):192–7.
55. LeBus GF, Collinge C. Vascular abnormalities as assessed with CT angiography in high-energy tibial plafond fractures. J Orthop Trauma 2008;22(1):16–22.
56. Patterson MJ, Cole JD. Two-staged delayed open reduction and internal fixation of severe pilon fractures. J Orthop Trauma 1999;13(2):85–91.
57. Sirkin M, Sanders R, DiPasquale T, et al. A staged protocol for soft tissue management in the treatment of complex pilon fractures. J Orthop Trauma 1999; 13(2):78–84.
58. Blauth M, Bastian L, Krettek C, et al. Surgical options for the treatment of severe tibial pilon fractures: a study of three techniques. J Orthop Trauma 2001;15(3): 153–60.
59. Bozic V, Thordarson DB, Hertz J. Ankle fusion for definitive management of nonreconstructable pilon fractures. Foot Ankle Int 2008;29(9):914–8.
60. Pollak AN, McCarthy ML, Bess RS, et al. Outcomes after treatment of high-energy tibial plafond fractures. J Bone Joint Surg Am 2003;85-A(10):1893–900.
61. Teeny SM, Wiss DA. Open reduction and internal fixation of tibial plafond fractures. Variables contributing to poor results and complications. Clin Orthop Relat Res 1993;(292):108–17.
62. Kline AJ, Gruen GS, Pape HC, et al. Early complications following the operative treatment of pilon fractures with and without diabetes. Foot Ankle Int 2009;30(11): 1042–7.
63. Zelle BA, Gruen GS, McMillen RL, et al. Primary arthrodesis of the tibiotalar joint in severely comminuted high-energy pilon fractures. J Bone Joint Surg Am 2014; 96(11):e91.
64. Hsu AR, Lareau CR, Anderson RB. Repair of acute superficial deltoid complex avulsion during ankle fracture fixation in National Football League players. Foot Ankle Int 2015;36(11):1272–8.
65. Niikura T, Miwa M, Sakai Y, et al. Ankle arthrodesis using antegrade intramedullary nail for salvage of nonreconstructable tibial pilon fractures. Orthopedics 2009;32(8):24–6.

Intramedullary Nailing of Fibular Fractures

Justin J. Fleming, DPM

KEYWORDS

• Intramedullary fixation • Fibular fracture repair • Malleolar fracture

KEY POINTS

- The reamed intramedullary (IM) technique has many benefits.
- Despite these many benefits, open plating is the technique most commonly used.
- In the past, IM stabilization was reserved for fibular fractures, which were given lower priority, and generally associated with injuries to the distal tibia or instances in which the soft tissue envelope was otherwise unsuitable for an open approach.

Level of Evidence: Level V, expert opinion.

Statically locked, reamed, intramedullary (IM) fixation has been mainstay of treatment in long bone fractures of the tibia and femur. This mode of fracture stabilization has multiple benefits, which include

- Minimally invasive insertion
- Soft tissue preservation
- Mechanically stable by placing fixation along the anatomic axis of the bone
- Load-sharing properties
- Axially and rotationally stable via interlocking screws
- Allowance for earlier weightbearing with controlled axial motion
- High union rates.

Despite these advantages, the mainstay of fibular fracture repair has been open plating. Perhaps this is due to a previous lack of dedicated anatomic IM implants and the knowledge that fibular length, rotation, and axial alignment are critical to mortise stability and long-term joint health. In the past, IM stabilization was reserved for fibular fractures, which were given lower priority, and generally associated with injuries to the distal tibia or instances in which the soft tissue envelope was otherwise unsuitable for an open approach. A renewed interest in this technique for primary fibular fractures, coupled with improved implants, has made this a viable treatment option for the foot and ankle surgeon.

Disclosure: Dr J.J. Fleming is a consultant for Arthrex Inc.
University Orthopaedic Associates, 2 World's Fair Drive, Somerset, NJ 08873, USA
E-mail address: flemingjmak@gmail.com

Clin Podiatr Med Surg 35 (2018) 259–270
https://doi.org/10.1016/j.cpm.2017.12.008

INDICATIONS FOR FIBULAR NAILING

The indications for this device are evolving with time and experience, but they have typically been used in clinical scenarios in which the conditions of the surrounding soft tissue envelope were suboptimal and/or the patient's medical comorbidities presented a significant risk. Current indications include

- Geriatric ankle fractures
- Fragility fractures
- Ankle fractures associated with peripheral vascular disease
- Diabetic ankle fractures
- Any soft tissue envelope compromised or in which intrinsic medical risk is elevated
- Tobacco use
- Poor compliance
- Advanced age
- High injury severity (fracture or dislocation and/or high energy mechanism).

The primary indication remains malleolar fractures in the geriatric population. The injuries are typically given a lower priority owing to technical difficulties with stabilization of porotic fractures; a designation that older patients are less active and, therefore, their treatment should be more conservative; and, finally, because the overwhelming body

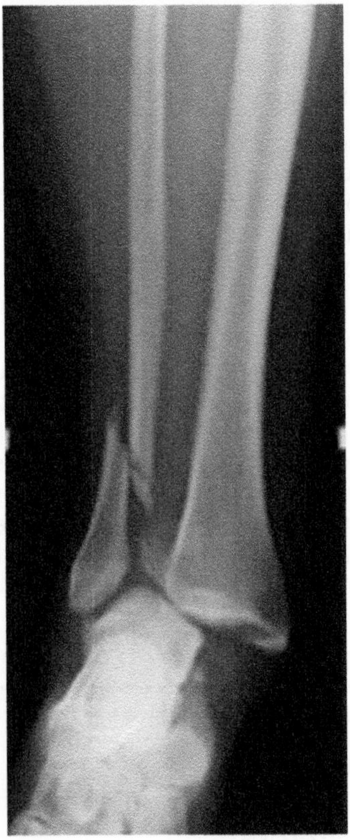

Fig. 1. PER 4 Fracture/Dislocation with significant ligamentous injury.

of literature demonstrates that these patients have a high incidence of wound complications, leading to poor outcomes. Surgical management of unstable ankle fractures in this population is critical to restoring skeletal stability and returning to ambulation, which is necessary for longevity and the prevention of secondary complications.

In the author's opinion, current relative contraindications include any rotational ankle fractures that possess a high ligament-to-bone injury ratio. This simply means that the ligamentous component is markedly greater than the fracture component. An example is a pronation external rotation (PER) 4 injury with complete syndesmotic injury disruption and a deltoid rupture (or anterior collicular fracture and deep deltoid combination as described by Tornetta) (**Fig. 1**). These injuries, if possible, are best treated through selective soft tissue reconstruction based on intraoperative stress examinations. Another area of concern is the insensate diabetic ankle fracture. Current thought is that these injuries are best treated with multiple transsyndesmotic screws used the tibia-pro-fibula approach (**Fig. 2**). Based on available nail designs, there are 2 positions for syndesmotic fixation. These may be inadequate if dense neuropathy exists coupled with significant instability patterns.

LITERATURE REVIEW

The body of literature is sparse but growing on the topic of fibular nailing. The recent studies can be divided into 2 broad categories: mechanical testing and clinical outcomes.

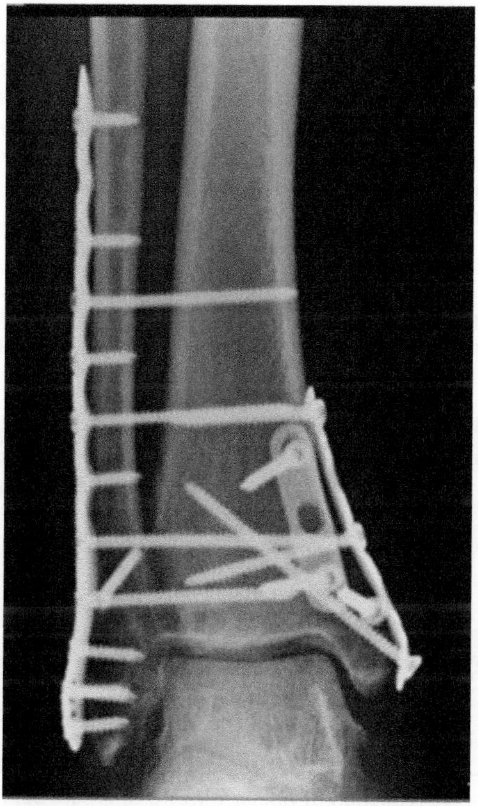

Fig. 2. Tibia-pro-fibula approach used for creating a superconstruct in the insensate patient.

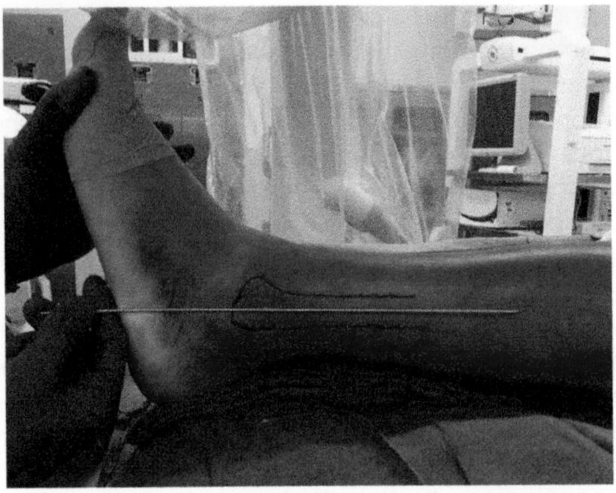

Fig. 3. Preoperative determination of the long axis of the fibula utilizing fluoroscopic guidance.

Mechanical Testing

Kadakia and colleagues[1] evaluated an external stress model in a PER 4 fracture pattern by comparing a laterally placed locking plate and an IM nail. Both fixation constructs had a single syndesmotic screw. Both cyclical loading and load to failure were performed. They concluded that there were no significant differences in rotatory strength with either form of fixation. All specimens failed at the level of the syndesmotic screw.

Oliver White and colleagues[2] performed similar testing in a supination external rotation IV model with a nonlocking neutralization plate or lag screw, and a dedicated IM nail. No syndesmotic screws were used and external rotation stress was performed to ultimate failure. Their results demonstrated greater torque to failure and better maintenance of the fibular construct for the IM fibular nail compared with standard plating.

Clinical Outcomes

In a study of 24 fragility fractures[3] treated with a locked fibular nail, no wound breakdown or deep infections developed at 1-year follow-up. The average subject age was

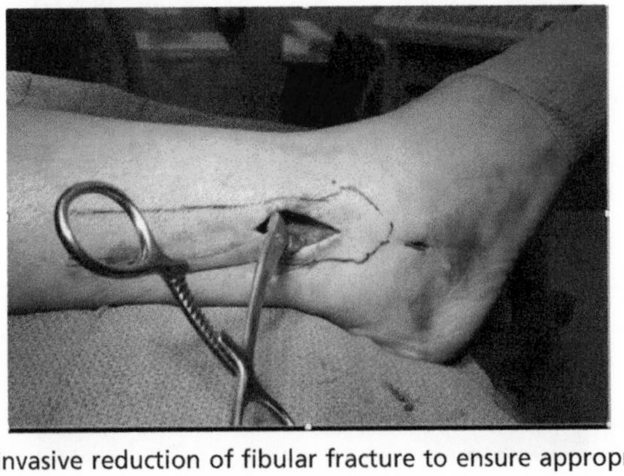

Fig. 4. Minimally invasive reduction of fibular fracture to ensure appropriate length, rotation and axial alignment.

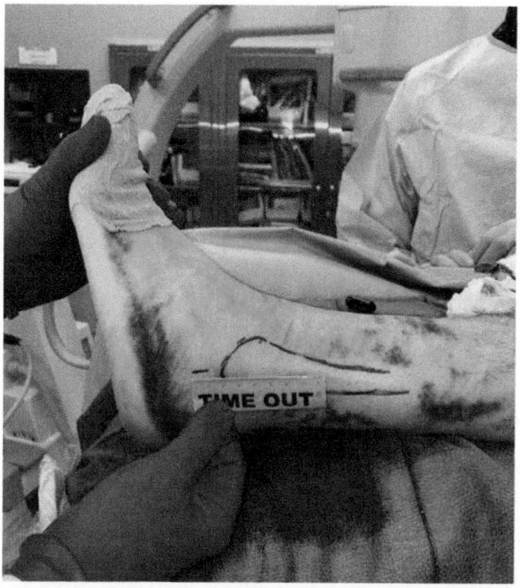

Fig. 5. Small vertical incision created beneath the inferior tip of the fibula.

79 years of age. They concluded that the use of fibular locking nails is "crucial to achieve early mobilization and also to maintain a good fracture position." They cited low complication rates, high patient satisfaction, and early return to function as significant benefits.

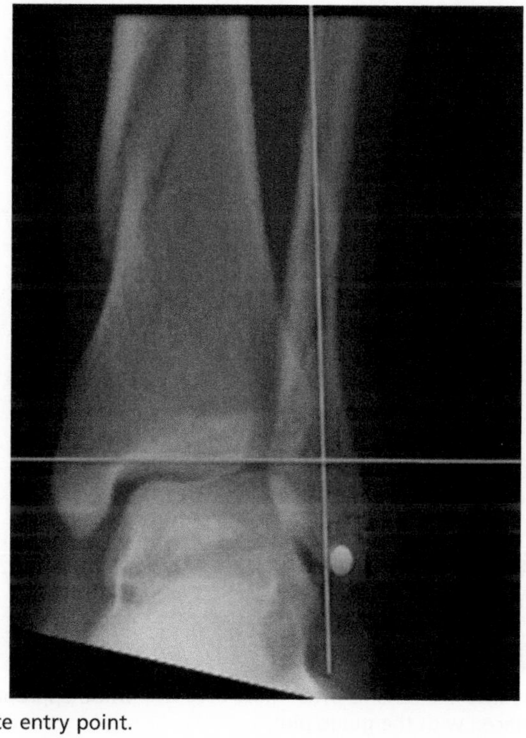

Fig. 6. Appropriate entry point.

A prospective randomized controlled trial of the fibular nail versus standard open reduction and internal fixation for fixation of ankle fractures in elderly subjects was published by Court-Brown and colleagues.[4] The primary measurement for outcome was the Olerud-Molander Ankle Score. Their results demonstrated no difference in functional recovery at 1 year between open plating and fibular nailing, with fewer soft tissue complications with IM fixation.

Brew and colleagues[5] performed a systemic review of IM fixation of unstable ankle fractures. They identified 17 studies with more than 1000 subjects. They found that "intramedullary fixation of unstable distal fibular fractures can give excellent results that are comparable with modern plating techniques. However, as yet, there is unconvincing evidence that it is superior to standard techniques with regards to clinical and functional outcomes."

OPERATIVE TECHNIQUE

The modified operative technique for the Fibulock fibular nail (Arthrex Inc, Naples, FL, USA) described herein is based on the author's clinical experience. First and foremost, anatomic fracture reduction is paramount regardless of the mode of stabilization. Although this may often be referred to as a percutaneous method, in the author's experience a small 2 to 3 cm incision is created to ensure adequate reduction. Less commonly, the fracture can be reduced percutaneously or become secondarily reduced following reduction of the medial sided injury.

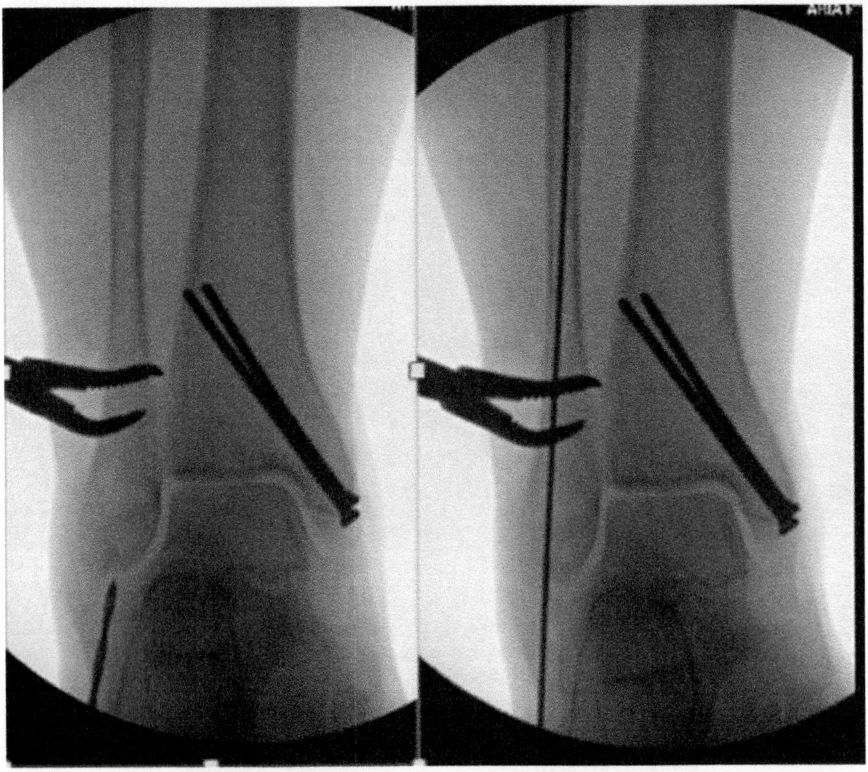

Fig. 7. Drill bit entry into the canal is often more accurate. Once the canal is identified the drill bit may be replaced with the guide pin.

As with any less invasive surgery, a greater appreciation of surface anatomy and increased use of fluoroscopy is helpful. Before surgical intervention a true lateral radiograph is obtained using the guide pin to identify the long axis of the fibula (**Fig. 3**).

The remainder of the procedure can be done mainly using the anteroposterior plane radiographically. After the fracture is reduced (**Fig. 4**), the nail insertion sequence can begin.

A small vertical incision is created beneath the inferior tip of the fibula (**Fig. 5**).

Blunt dissection will quickly lead the inferior cortex of the fibula. Using a mortise view, a crosshair is imagined overlying the distal fibula. The appropriate entry point or so-called sweet spot is just lateral to the midline (**Fig. 6**).

A 2.5-mm drill bit is used to breach the cortex and find the IM canal.

The author relies on the drill bit instead of the guide pin for several reasons. The drill bit is side-cutting and can be steered to the appropriate direction without significant deformation. The tactile feel of the drill bit is superior to a smooth guide pin. Also, if the entry point is missed, a drill bit makes the creation of an adjacent entry point easier and more efficient. After the drill bit is within the canal, it can be exchanged through the drill guide for the cannulated guide pin (**Fig. 7**).

The distal end of the fibular metaphysis and canal are dilated with a 6.2-mm reamer followed by a 3.2-mm reamer to complete the step, allowing appropriate nail or endosteal fit (**Fig. 8**).

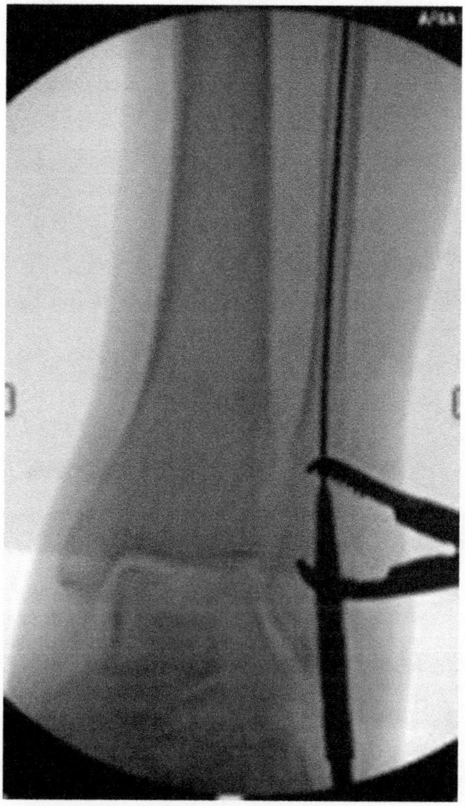

Fig. 8. Dilation of the distal fibula with 6.2 mm reamer.

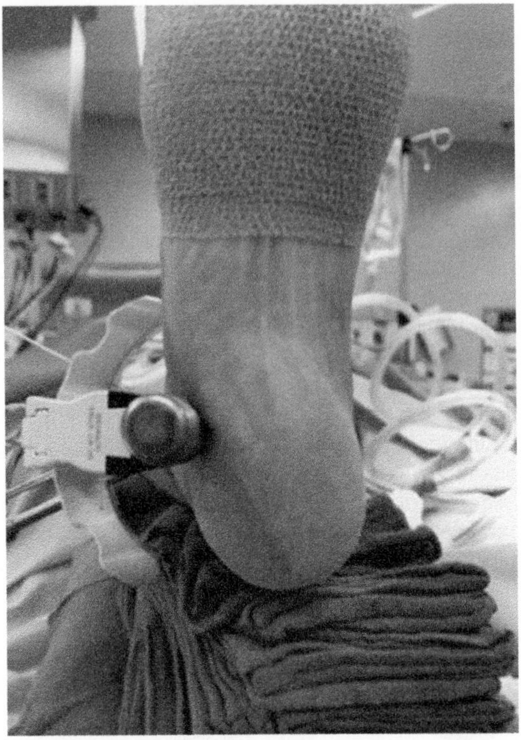

Fig. 9. Placement of the towel bump will allow for unaltered postion of targeting guide and ultimately appropriate angle for syndesmotic stabilization.

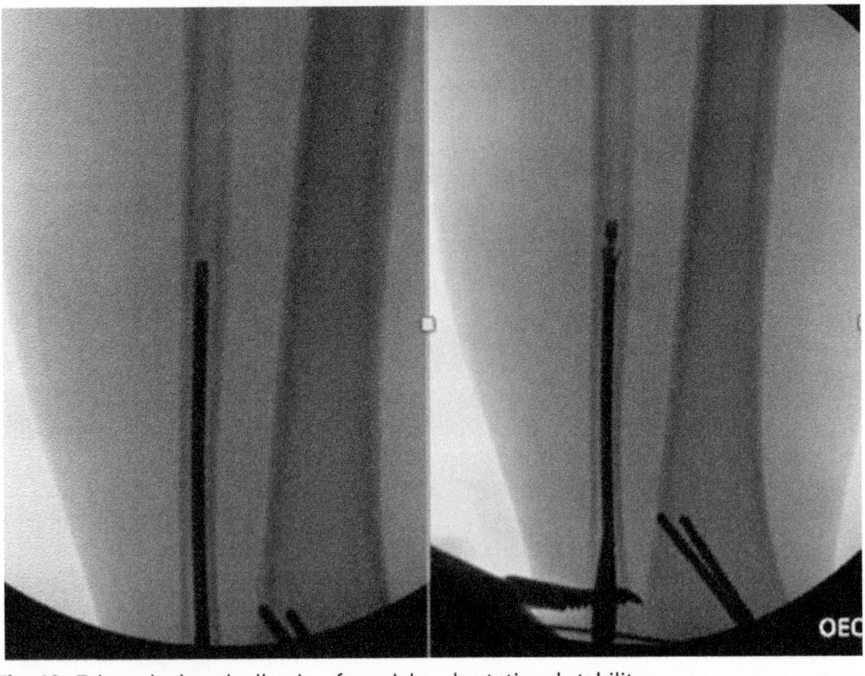

Fig. 10. Talons deployed, allowing for axial and rotational stability.

One potential pitfall may occur if the entry point is laterally placed. This will place the lateral cortex at risk during initial reaming. The nail may then be inserted using the jig to help guide its path under fluoroscopic guidance. Important details include making sure that the nail is slightly countersunk in the distal fibula and that the most distal syndesmotic hole is at or above the physeal scar of the tibia. If it is not, it may preclude this point of transsyndesmotic stabilization. It is also necessary to access nail rotation because this determines the appropriate angle of endobutton or screw fixation. The jig targets the nail at the level of the syndesmotic hole with a predetermined 30-degree offset to mimic the bimalleolar axis. Malrotation of the nail will affect this angle and potentially the reduction of the syndesmosis. Placement of a towel bump beneath the ankle will prevent the jig from coming into contact with the table and assist in targeting (**Fig. 9**).

The jig may be secured to the tibia with a K-wire to maintain alignment. Fracture reduction is again assessed visually and fluoroscopically. The talons may then be deployed, allowing for axial and rotational stability (**Fig. 10**).

The multidirectional targeted interlocking screws may then be inserted into the distal fibula though the jig. These screws typically range from 16 to 20 mm in length. The single antirotational wire may be removed and an external rotation stress test may be performed. If positive, the syndesmosis is stabilized with an endobutton device and retested. Persistent instability may require increased tensioning of the endobutton, the addition of

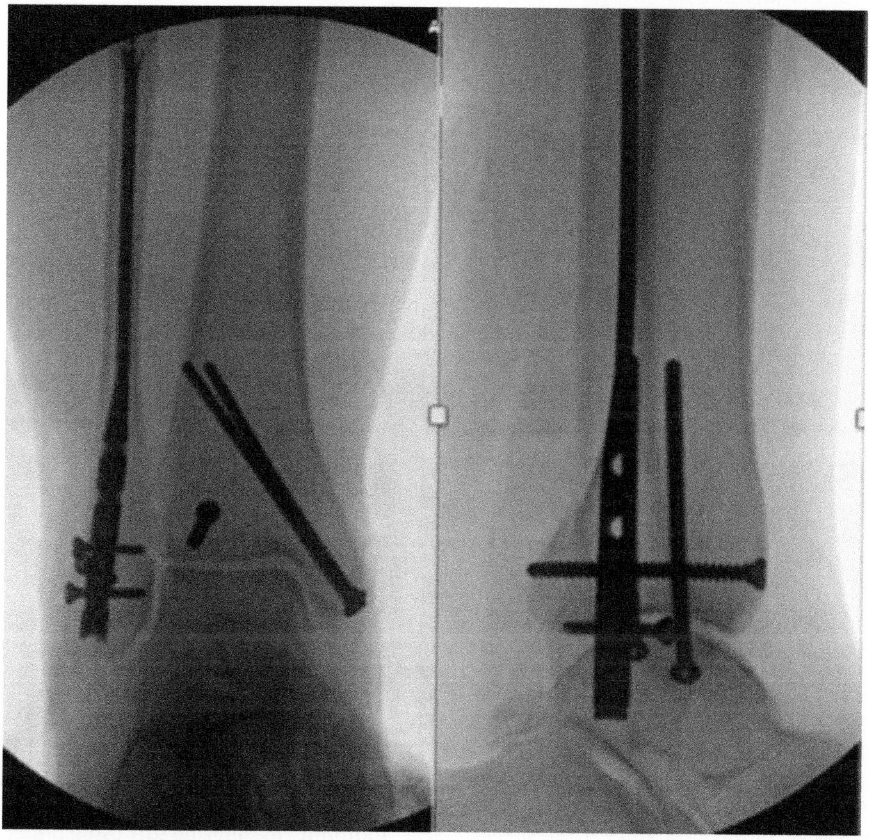

Fig. 11. Final intraoperative films.

a second endobutton, and/or the use of polyethylene suture to reconstruct the anterior syndesmotic ligaments. After the syndesmosis has satisfactory reduction or stability, a valgus stress test is performed to evaluate whether repair of the deltoid ligament is necessary. An end cap is available and used based on surgeon preference (**Fig. 11**).

CASE EXAMPLES

1. A 74-year-old woman sustained a closed insufficiency fracture of the distal tibia or fibula secondary to a mechanical fall. Single-stage surgical treatment consisted of closed reduction and provisional placement of a simple pin-to-bar construct. Following satisfactory alignment, the fibular fracture was repaired with IM nail. The tibia component was stabilized in minimally invasive fashion with a distally locked medial distal tibial plate (**Fig. 12**). The utilization of these techniques reduced the surgical footprint, preserved the blood supply to the injured structures, and minimized surgical risk for this patient. Protected weightbearing began at approximately 4 weeks.
2. A 36-year-old patient with insulin-dependent diabetes mellitus sustained an open grade 3 tibial plafond fracture with an associated fibular shaft fracture. He had a hemoglobin A1C value of 10.6. He was immediately placed in the open fracture protocol and was brought to the operating room for a washout, debridement, and skeletal stabilization. Based on his sustained elevated glucose levels, IM fixation of the lateral column was chosen. Following closed reduction and placement of a medially based external fixator, the fibular fracture was reduced by percutaneous methods and a fibular nail was introduced. Two weeks later, the tibial component was reconstructed through an anterolateral approach (**Fig. 13**).

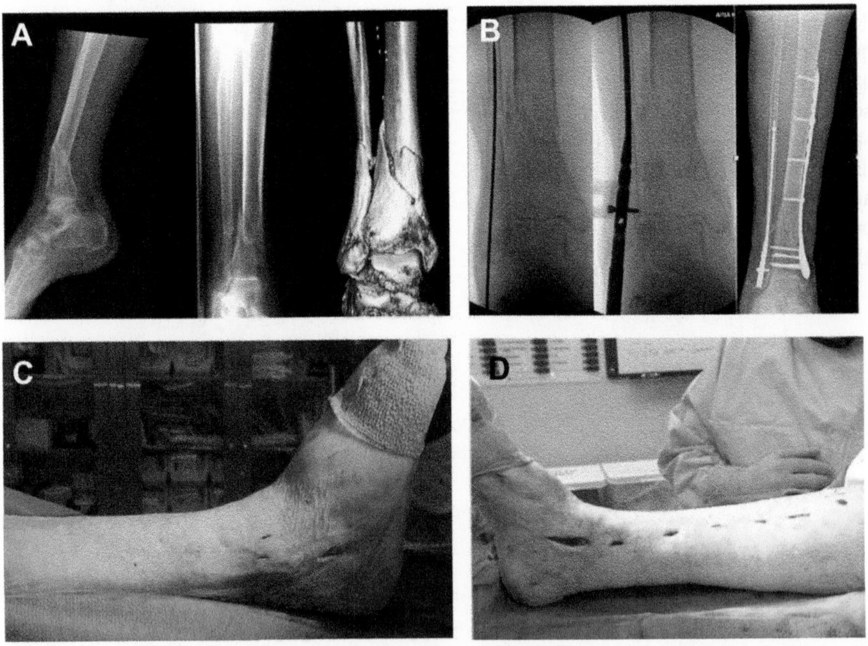

Fig. 12. (*A*) Low energy closed geriatric insufficiency fracture of the tibia and fibula. (*B*) Closed reduction and percuanteous stabilization ultizing an intramedulalry fibular nail and MIPO of the distal tibia. (*C, D*) Small surgical "footprint" maximizing soft tissue preservation and minimizing surgical risk.

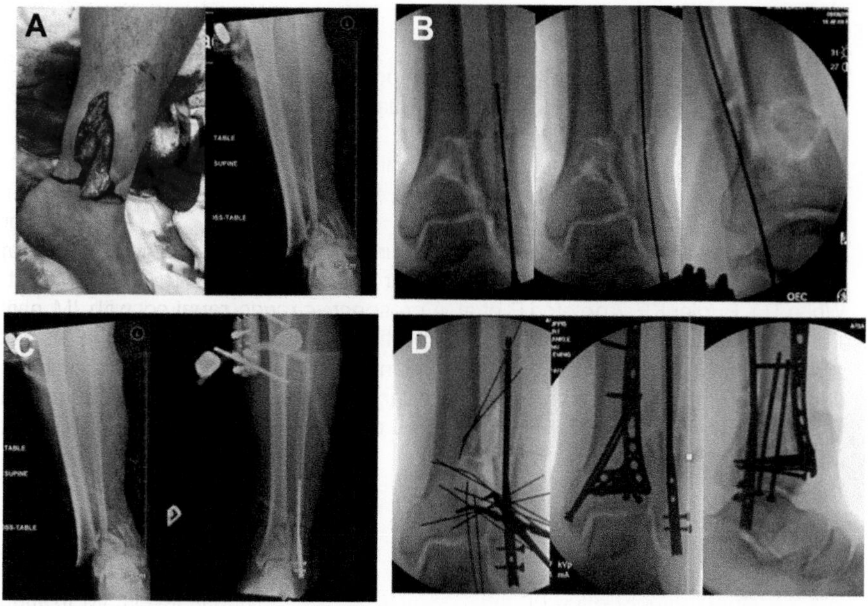

Fig. 13. (*A–C*) Stage 1 of fracture stabilization including minimally invasive placement of fibular nail and placement of external fixator. (*D*) Tibial component reconstructed through an anterolateral approach.

SUMMARY

IM nailing is a useful method to stabilize fractures of the fibula. Second-generation designs of the Fibulock nail allow for axial or rotation stability with fixed angle distal interlocking screws achieving construct strength similar to screw or plate fixation (**Fig. 14**). Based on current studies, this seems to be a safe and effective management tool in select populations. Patients with high-risk incisions due to a poor soft tissue envelope, especially those of advanced age, or significant medical comorbidities, may benefit from this technique because it reduces wound complications and shortens the duration of postoperative convalescence.

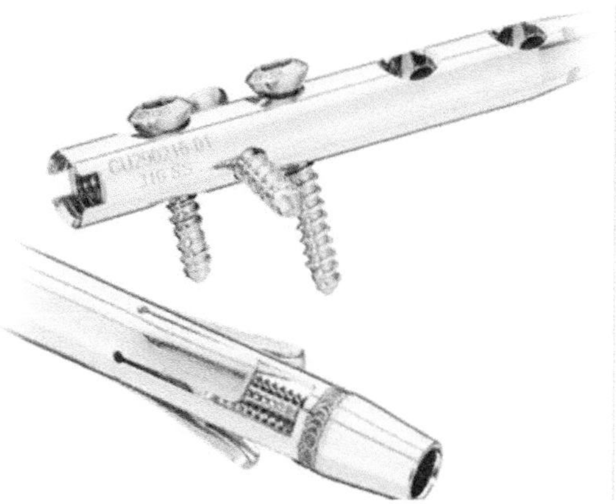

Fig. 14. Fibulock features. (These images were provided *courtesy of* Arthrex, Inc. 2017.)

REFERENCES

1. Witaj PJ, Fuchs D, Alshouli M, et al. A biomechanical comparison study of a modern fibular nail and distal fibular locking plate in AO/OTA 44c2 ankle fractures. J Orthop Surg Res 2016;11(1):100.
2. Smith G, Mackenzie SP, Wallace RJ, et al. Biomechanical comparison of intramedullary fibular nail versus plate and screw fixation. Foot Ankle Int 2017;38(12):1394–9.
3. Rajeev A, Senevirathna S, Radha S, et al. Functional outcomes after fibula locking nail for fragility fractures of the ankle. J Foot Ankle Surg 2011;50(5):547–50.
4. White TO, Bugler KE, Appleton P, et al. A prospective randomised controlled trial of the fibular nail versus standard open reduction and internal fixation for fixation of ankle fractures in elderly patients. Bone Joint J 2016;98-B(9):1248–52.
5. Jain S, Haughton BA, Brew C. Intramedullary fixation of distal fibular fractures: a systematic review of clinical and functional outcomes. J Orthop Traumatol 2014;15(4):245–54.

Printed and bound by CPI Group (UK) Ltd, Croydon, CR0 4YY
03/10/2024
01040395-0012